Beauty and the Yeast Beast:
From Fat to Fairy Tale

Francine Hemway

FIRST EDITION

Library of Congress Cataloging-in-Publication Data
Hemway, Francine
Beauty and the Yeast Beast: From Fat to Fairy Tale
By Francine Hemway – 1st Ed

ISBN 0-9786234-0-1
$39.95 Soft cover
1. Diet 2. Nutrition

Preface
Unwilling Obesity is a Disease

Francine Hemway wrote this book not as a survivor, but as a conqueror who, through tenacity, understanding, and self diagnostics, beat the Yeast Beast. Writing a blueprint for success as she developed and discovered the basic secrets of the connection between Yeast and obesity, and her articulation of the workings of this connection and how to combat it distinguishes Francine Hemway as an icon of life control. This book is meant for those suffering in silence, and for those who share their suffering, not knowing why, or how to help.

The Yeast Beast is exposed and the conquest of the Yeast Beast made practical by this book and journal. For the many sufferers of unwanted weight gain, unwilling obesity, and the yo-yo dieting of weight loss, this guide will bring about rationality and understanding. The *why* of uncontrolled weight gain and failure, of the many attempts at getting weight under control leading to Diet Failure Syndrome are now understandable. Those involved in this frustrating and maddening morass of the embarrassing, *"Why can't I/he/she get control?"* no longer have to feel guilty. The question of, *"Why didn't all the doctors and weight loss programs work?"* can now be answered for many. This is not just another diet book; it is a definitive solution to chronic and morbid unwilling obesity.

Obesity is a National problem, one person at a time.

Table of Contents

Introduction

Six years ago, when I turned forty-nine, I realized I would turn fifty in a year: half a century of life gone by with an undetermined amount to go. I was over 308 pounds (last recorded weight, and a size 26), tired, moody, sometimes antagonistic, often ornery or critical, and concerned about my long term, later-age health.

Over the last six years, several unrelated instances serendipitously converged, leading to the piecing together of a radical shift in my understanding of my weight problems and to the ability to overcome them. I learned how to lose the weight, keep it off, and face the *Curse of the Yeast Beast*. I learned what the Yeast Beast is, and how it works to keep us fat, to keep our attempts at permanent weight loss futile, despite allowing us intermittent successes.

In this introduction I simply want to capsulate the past and chronicle the factors that were prominent in these changes to give you a broad overview of where I was, where I am now, how I got here, and what I learned that rescued my life.

The book first introduces the sinister workings of the Yeast Beast (Candida), both biologically and psychologically. It also presents information on aging and obesity; not growing old obese is most likely the best and most pertinent reason existing for finally getting the Yeast Beast under control and bringing your weight to a healthy level. It explains the problem and the solution path: Yeast control, diet and (although optional, highly recommended) exercise. If you suffer in any way from being overweight, or care about someone who does, this section of the book will without doubt shed new light on an old problem. The book then explains what I did, what I had to learn (and to face) and offers explanation of those things you are probably going to have to do, and learn (and face). Long term weight problems/obesity is a harsh subject; there are some harsh truths contained in this book.

The journal provides a place for data tracking and journaling opportunities which will help you get a more complete picture of where you are and how you are progressing; it offers tips and encouragement. While completing the journal is optional, in retrospect it becomes a valuable tool and I highly suggest that you utilize it; if you are one of those folks like me who hates to put things down in writing *just in case*, let me just say that looking back, I know I would have made fewer mistakes and have learned more about myself sooner if I'd have had available and kept a journal such as this.

I am not a medical doctor or a health professional, and I offer no medical advice. This book contains important information about the *Yeast Beast* and the *Curse of the Yeast Beast* for those who are long term, seriously overweight or obese and those who are close to them. This program worked for me; I lost 180 pounds and have kept it off for five years. If you would like to pursue the Phasing Program outlined in this book, you should contact your physician first.

I just blew up.

I was a skinny little tot. There's a picture of me at three climbing on a swing, wearing my Patty Play Pal doll's clothes, which are falling off of me. My mother says when I turned five I just 'blew up'. She offers no explanation for this, though in this book I offer some relative theories.

My memory doesn't go back far enough to remember a time I wasn't grossly overweight for my age, despite being tall. In the sixth grade I was 5'6¾ " tall and weighed 135. While on the health charts this is not overweight, the charts are calibrated for adults; I was not an adult. I was twelve years old, and weighed a good forty to fifty pounds more than any of the other girls in the school. In high school my weight was in the 180's; I was still 5'6¾ ". (I'm now 5'5".)

As far back as I can remember, my parents told people my older sister was the pretty one, the beauty, and I was the smart one, the brain. In retrospect, it did me double harm. It programmed me that I was not pretty, and it made me over-focus on my smarts, and to use my brain as a defensive mechanism; it set me up with an unconscious concept that, as the old T-shirt sports:

"I May Be Fat, But You're Stupid.
I can always lose weight."

I was a tomboy and somewhat athletic, though I never played sports formally. Looking back, I think if I hadn't been too embarrassed to wear shorts or a swim suit or to run in public, I might have been a lot more athletic. I rode my bike a lot growing up, and, when I got into high school and bikes just weren't cool, I walked a lot. I worked for a veterinarian while I was in high school where I would frequently and easily picked up sixty-five plus pound dogs and lifted them onto the examining table. So I was always strong, despite being overweight.

I'd lost weight several times along the way. I joined Weight Watchers in high school, and met with moderate success, but it was short lived. I was very successful with Atkins once, and went down to a size fourteen, the smallest I ever got on any diet in my life prior to discovering the Yeast Beast, but any return to a normal food selection– even adding a piece of fresh fruit to my regimen– brought about a return of the weight along with additional poundage and, as I later learned, a reduction of muscle.

I read every diet book that came out, and have time logged with varying success on Atkins, Pritikin, South Beach, Grapefruit diet, Liquid Protein Diet, Slim-Fast, Dr. Phil's Diet, Fit for Life, The Zone, Sugar Busters, and have been through appetite suppressants, a medical program with a 500 calorie diet and daily injections, the hypnotism, the acupuncture, laser therapy; if it was a diet or treatment program with any exposure between 1961, when I started dieting as a ten year old, until 2001, when I turned fifty and reached a weight loss (then) of 168 pounds, I had read it, tried it, and met with incomplete and unable-to-maintain results. I can cite at least twenty-three separate, serious dieting phases in my thirty-five years of obesity. Between the diet books I've read and the research I've done on line, I have logged more hours on learning diets than I did to obtain my Masters Degree. If a PhD. was available in Weight Loss and Dieting, I'd have earned it.

All diets work once
you learn to
control the Yeast Beast.

The first of several serendipitous events was the suggestion by Elaine, my health care provider, a knowledgeable, dedicated, and extremely sharp nurse who was my doctor's assistant, that I get tested for Candida, a Yeast that causes numerous health issues; she felt that, in addition to my weight issues, my tired, moody, and various other issues could be related to a Yeast infestation. As a side note, I had been treated by a highly competent urologist for two years with DMSO infusions internally for interstitial cystitis, a bladder disease; the treatments were fairly ineffective. Once the Yeast was controlled, **_all_** symptoms of the interstitial cystitis disappeared.

Elaine recommended I read and follow *The Schwartzbein Principle.* I began a diet completely devoid of sugar and starch and highly processed foods for two weeks, planning to follow Dr. Schwartzbein's diet. I took Grapefruit Seed Extract to help reduce the Yeast, and acidophilus to bolster beneficial microbes. Elaine prescribed Nystatin as well; Nystatin is a prescription drug which is effective against Yeast overgrowth, but I was unable to tolerate it. I later learned about and utilized other anti-fungals and additional probiotics. I also learned the importance of alternating them. These are both are discussed later in the book.

The second, closely related event was that Elaine sent me to a Chinese Medicine specialist, who did food allergy testing; I learned I was allergic to sugar (both beet and cane), white and wheat flour, chocolate, cocoa, corn, and soy. I learned we acquire food allergies by overloading our systems with those foods we are allergic to, and that we *crave* what we're allergic to, which contributes to the overloading. It's a vicious cycle, a "Which came first, the chicken or the egg?"

The Yeast Beast actually makes you Crave sugar, flour, and starches; that's what it likes and needs to live on.

When I returned to the doctor's two weeks later, I'd lost over ten pounds and was feeling more energetic, more focused, and less moody. I stayed on the restrictive part of the diet for almost four years after the Yeast had been controlled because I felt good, and it had served me well to lose 168 pounds and keep it off. I was terrified of regaining the weight. I splurged when I wanted to, but immediately returned to the protein diet, afraid a return to normal food groups on a daily basis would result in a loss of control over my weight; had I known what I know now, I could have moved to a less restrictive, more nutritionally balanced diet much sooner. Today I eat everything, just not all the time, not as much as I could, and not without working for it.

The next fortuitous event was the gift for my fiftieth birthday of a fourteen year old retired cow pony, Jake, who became a source of exercise and led to the decision to take a year off from education (I was a public school superintendent) to break and train horses. We trained and sold twenty-four horses that year, and at one point had ten horses at one time; I was doing a lot of feeding, grooming, schooling (arena, mountain, desert, and beach training), and hiking back and forth to the corrals. At fifty years old, I was starting to build the first signs of muscle strength I'd seen since I was a teenager. I also lost more weight.

Time came to return to work, and we moved to another county; we only took with us the three horses I had gentle-broke and trained as two year olds. Things in my marriage had been strained for some time, though I was in denial about this, and the divorce was not something I had seen coming nor wanted. My perspective on these events now is much different, and much closer to the truth, than that at the time. It was only after obesity recovery and rehab began that I was able to see the ways in which I'd contributed to inter-personal difficulties in my life, not only in my marriage, but with my family and those I worked for and with.

I considered accepting a superintendency in Northern California, but my mother was very ill with COPD and it was good for her and for me that I instead move to Florida to be with her and help her. She was hospitalized several times that winter, and I ran a three month bout with a sore throat that would not go away; then we discovered she had a serious mold problem in the house. My mother went to stay in Miami with my older sister and the contractor and mold remediator went to work. Almost a month later, when they could not get the house to clear, serendipity blessed me again; they called in the foremost expert in the mold field: Edward.

It was a difficult infestation, complicated by some contractor mistakes that actually inadvertently worked to *provide* an inviting growth environment for the mold, and it took a few weeks remediate the house, but it finally cleared. My mother has not had any recurrence of the repeated hospitalizations since the mold was cleared; while she still has severe COPD, she can again live unassisted.

In the process of Edward's working to discover the source of the continued infestation, I became interested in mold and asked Edward to train me. I was very interested in the microbiology; actually, when I was in high school I was a Biology geek and had always planned and expected to move into the sciences when I went to college.

I had begun daily walking two years ago when I moved to Florida. The depression from the divorce, being out of work, and having my day center around my mother's needs (including marathon sleeping events due to her weakened condition) left me pretty much a couch potato; walking replaced the horse exercise, though was much less effective overall. I found the walking gave me personal space (and I walked at 4 AM so there was not even anyone out there to have to acknowledge with a perfunctory 'Hi'.) I also found it helped with the depression to walk. As I challenged myself to move from one mile a day to two, and then to the two miles a day in an hour, and then to forty minutes, I began to look forward to this time for me. I realized that taking time to do things for me – not the errands and needs, but time for me, for my mental and physical health – was something I had never learned to do.

Edward and I walked a lot during the weeks he worked on the house; we walked for hours. We could talk and he could teach about the kinds of molds, how they grew, how to recover them from the environment, and how to propagate them for identification; it all fascinated me. The long days and evenings working at my mother's apartment had been keeping him from his normal, and serious, daily workout schedule at home, so we walked, and we walked, and we walked.

Edward suggested I add ankle and wrist weights on my legs and arms. While they were awkward at first, it was not difficult, and the benefits of adding weights evidenced quickly; I began to drop the twelve pounds that had crept up during the actual divorce process (which had me very paranoid, and I was much relieved to see them go), and I could feel the beginnings (the very beginnings) of some muscle firming. I returned to a size six; as I increased the amount of weight I carried and the length of my stride and swing during my walks, I dropped down to a size four.

Now a certified and licensed Mold Inspector and Remediator, I opened *Florida Institute of Mold* with Edward's help and guidance. We soon became business partners. Because we spent so much time together, Edward got to know me very well; actually, I realized later, he had gotten to know me much better than I knew myself. I had difficulty understanding the problems he had with me, both physically and psychologically, and he had a lot of problems with me; I could not see me as he did. He probably spent almost as much time talking to me about what was wrong with me as he did about mold. He told me the story of the old witch, which I will share with you a little later in the book; this story made a huge contribution to my mental attitude regarding diet and exercise (or no-exercise), and how I wanted things to be as I moved on in future years.

The next huge serendipitous occurrence was a conversation Edward and I had about my weight loss, lifetime diet history, and Elaine's hitting the nail on the head about the Candida. Molds are members of the family of Fungi, and so are Yeast. Both are part of the fabric of life. Yeast resides within us normally and commensally (of, relating to, or characterized by a symbiotic relationship in which one species is benefited while the other is unaffected). I never knew this.

I learned a lot about Fungi from Edward, and from reading two books he recommended: Larone's *Medically Important Fungi* and Barnett and Hunter's *Illustrated Genera of Imperfect Fungi*. Because of my involvement in mold, I was able to see and finally understand the microbiology of what had happened to me. Because of the information I shared with Edward, he was able to make some important, relevant scientific connections. For the first time I began to look at Candida not as some labeled parasite that I had acquired and gotten rid of and then afterwards stayed on that diet because it was helping me to lose weight, but as a living entity, a distinct life form, normal to my system in measured amounts which had grown completely out of control under one of the environmental situations which provide the perfect conditions for vigorous growth, an entity which actually *caused* the weight gain. My body had been invaded from within.

There is no *getting rid of* Yeast, merely the ability to keep it at bay. Yeast is, literally, an opportunistic, vicious, and unrelenting Beast which has plagued me since childhood, keeping me obese despite all efforts and intermittent successes, affecting my whole life, and every personal and professional relationship I had in ways I, nor my family, could understand.

Around this time, Edward worked on grooming me, as his partner, for business. As a public school administrator, I had many cross–over skills, but was missing some important skills relating to the workings of the mold business and that service industry. I was also, in hindsight, deficient in the presentation I made in appearance and demeanor. While as a school administrator there were of course times I was expected to dress up, I worked in small, rural districts and my usual attire was very casual; in hindsight, it was often almost sloppy. I rarely wore makeup, and my hair was always cut for wash-and-run; I had no time, nor talent, for it. I used to tell myself I was cosmetically retarded. (Be careful what you tell yourself; the mind hears what you say and takes it as gospel whether it is true or not.)

Of all the serendipitous events, I am most grateful for Edward deciding that I was worth it as a partner to deal with the rest of me as he saw it, and the long stream of insights he gave me and prodding he was willing to do to pursue this end. It was Edward who saw and articulated the *Curse of the Yeast Beast*, and supported me in pursuing physical conditioning, surgical constructive assistance to remove excess skin, and 'psychic surgery': the facing of the devastation of the battle with the Yeast Beast upon my body, my personality, and my life.

As Yeast phases from one form to another throughout its reproductive life cycle, so have I phased through different stages in my war with the Yeast Beast and the *Curse of the Yeast Beast*. Edward and I are now partners in marriage as well as business. He continues to support me as I continue to phase, and is as much responsible for the writing of this book as I am; I am grateful to him for both.

Chapter 1
Advanced Infirmation

The reality of our own mortality hits us some time in our thirties; we realize we won't live forever, and we recognize that people are living longer than they did fifty years ago. Some toss it off in a cavalier manner, a few go death-scare crazy; most are somewhere in the middle with me, getting it that we don't have forever, and consoling ourselves with the fact that we have longer.

I decided when I was forty-nine that I needed to shed the weight now or face for certain debilitating health issues when I aged: knee problems, arthritis, (try moving three hundred pounds out of bed when everything hurts), heart or other organ problems from the stress of the extra weight, diabetes (type II usually results from obesity), etc.

> ## *Advanced Infirmation is the process of increasingly developing new illness as you age more rapidly than normal due to obesity.*

When I moved to Florida to be with my mother, I found myself transported from small communities in rural areas of California, working with young teachers and younger parents and children, to a megalopolis, for me, of a city, Delray Beach, in a *single housing development* of more than 12,000 over fifty-five years old residents. (There are more people in this one development than in many of the cities I have lived in.) Most of these people bought these condos decades ago; the majority of the population here is over seventy-five, and most of them are in their eighties and nineties. I want you to know Bette Davis was being *subtle* when she said, "*Old age: it's not for sissies.*"

We see people here on a daily basis who need assistance or devices to get around: aides, walkers, wheelchairs, canes; we see folks on oxygen, as their circulation or lung capacity or heart strength impairs their ability to get air. We see not so old people, the 'young' crowd in their sixties, who are already obese, sedentary, and heading for all of the health problems associated with Geriatric Obesity.

Restaurants are full of people conversing about their sciatica, diabetes, blood pressure, edema (water retention), fatigue; the list is long, and the same conversations are overheard everywhere we go, coming from new strangers. People converse regarding their multiple medications, with varying directions on times to take them being confusing; they fear taking too many of something or not enough of something else. Many are taking so many something's, I worry that they suffer drug interactions they are not even aware of. I imagine that these might even present to a doctor as new symptoms, and yet another drug will be prescribed.

There are a few people who walk here, but it is mostly the 'young' sixties crowd; the majority of folks here get no more movement in a day than dressing and undressing, and going out to the clubhouse to play cards or take a ceramics class, or go shopping, *if* they go out at all. Many are quite housebound. Most are overweight. Most consume very large quantities of breads and sweets, and pre-packaged, over-processed foods and meals. If boxed sugar cereals and the TV dinner were an affront to good nutrition when I was five, bagels, Danish, and the microwave dinner have got to be an affront to good nutrition for the golden years.

There are three commodities you can not buy: love, health, and time. But you can invest in them now, and bank away for tomorrow.

Invest money in the bank, time in your loved ones, and energy in exercise

for your future health.

If you do a WWW search on obesity and health, you will come up with thousands of sites. (Yahoo returned 27,400,000 listings.) Among other ailments, obesity is listed as increasing a person's risk of illness and death due to diabetes, stroke, coronary artery disease, hypertension, high cholesterol, and kidney or gallbladder disorders; it may increase the risk for some types of cancer, and is also a risk factor for the development of osteoarthritis and sleep apnea (a condition in which one stops breathing in one's sleep for brief moments in time; an apnea incident can be fatal).

I belong to the Baby Boomer generation. In 2005, the Census Bureau put out a special statistics report. The following statistics come from this report:

In 2006, the oldest of the baby boomers, the generation born between1946 and 1964, will turn 60 years old.

78.2 million
Estimated number of baby boomers, as of July 1, 2005.

7,918
Number of people turning 60 each day in 2006, according to projections. That amounts to 330 every hour.

50.8%
Percentage of women baby boomers in 2005.

$2,695
Average annual expenditures on health care in 2004 for people ages 45 to 54 — the age group that is the heart of the baby boom generation. When budgeting medical expenses, baby boomers should expect increased health-care spending as they age; for instance, those aged 55 to 64 spent $3,262 and those 65 and over, $3,899.

57.8 million
Number of baby boomers living in 2030, according to projections; 54.9 percent would be female. That year, boomers would be between ages 66 and 84.

The Future: 4,041
Number of continuing care retirement facilities in 2003. Many boomers could

have parents in need of such facilities or may have to move into such a facility themselves in the future.

Yeast lives in the crevices of the digestive system, and on external portions of our body. But Yeast is mucoidal, and viscerous; it is just plain slimy. When you put filamentous fungal mold on a piece of tape and tape it to the slide, it stays there. When you try to get the tape with Yeast to adhere to the slide, the Yeast often just slips out between the slide and the tape. Just as cockroaches can get through anything because they have no bones, the near liquid state of many Yeast allow them to slither around your body freely and, as they are only one or two microns wide (there are 24,500 microns to an inch), the body doesn't detect them.

Yeast sets up home in adipose body fat (under the skin) and visceral fat (along the outside of organs) as easily as it does the gastrointestinal tract. When it sets up home in the bloodstream, you may develop a systemic infestation.

Yeast has access to every organ and system in your body, and as Yeast thrives and grows larger in you, greater amounts toxins are being released into your body, including Acetaldehyde, the toxin responsible for most of the symptoms you get when you have a hangover. Little wonder there are so many ailments attributed to Yeast. Many of these ailments lead to various degrees of infirmity.

We coined the phrase *advanced infirmation* to refer to the process of increasingly developing new illness as you age more rapidly than normal due to obesity.

I promised earlier to relate the story of the old witch. It goes like this:

> One day, a beautiful young witch was walking through the forest, when she came upon an elderly, stooped, and crooked couple in ragged clothing, looking for berries, as they had no food. She saw that despite their poverty and sad physical condition, they were still very much in love.

> She decided to give them a gift; she would make them young again, and they could relive their lives, making better decisions and earning more success, so that when they got old again they could enjoy their love in comfort.

> Some many years later, the witch, now an old witch, was walking through the woods when she once again came upon the couple. To

her surprise and dismay, they were again stooped, and crooked, in ragged clothing, looking for berries, as they had no food.

How can this be? She thought. *I gave you your whole lives over, and here you are, just as before.*

This story comes to my mind often. I look at what I do vigilantly to assure that down the road I will not find myself back as I used to be.

The message of this chapter is the most important message in the book:

<u>Obesity is slow suicide.</u>

No matter when you start, a healthy lifestyle improves your quality of life and may extend your lifespan. People who are physically active, eat healthily, avoid tobacco and alcohol, and who get regular check-ups are more likely to look forward to many years of staying active and independent than those of us who deviate from this regimen by varying degrees.

More than fifty percent of people die from preventable diseases, such as heart disease, cancer and stroke. How a body ages is linked in part to family patterns of aging and genetics, but the greatest impact on how well we age is made by our personal health behaviors. Our daily lifestyle choices have the most influence on how well, or poorly, our body ages, and what *quality of life* we have when we are old.

Choose an exercise you like and stick with it. Regular exercise is even more important for seniors than other age groups. Their risk of disease and lost mobility is greater. Look for ways every day to exercise in work and play. Stretch and walk whenever possible. Studies have been done which show that even sedentary people in their nineties can build muscle.

Don't think you need to run out and buy exercise suits and join a gym; in fact, if you're over fifty pounds overweight don't even think about an exercise program at all – just think about starting to re-awaken your muscles. Later in the book the whole issue of exercise/no-exercise is discussed in much more detail.

Exercise your mind by reading, learning a new skill, or researching something that interests you. The greatest enemy to the mind is depression; the greatest cause of depression is stagnation. Research shows that senior citizens who maintain hobbies or take on learning new skills suffer less depression and less dementia.

Chronic illnesses such as heart disease and cancer are having a greater impact on an increasingly aging population. Mental and neurological illnesses, such as depression and Alzheimer's disease, are more common in older adults. According to the Good Health Practices Study, a fifteen year study of more than 6900 people, researchers identified seven health habits that were good predictors of how long people lived. People following five or more of these health practices lived as much as eleven years longer than those following three or less:

1. Regular aerobic exercise (at least 30 minutes 3x/week)

2. Moderate alcohol use only

3. A good night's sleep

4. Maintaining a recommended body weight

5. Eating a good breakfast daily

6. Avoiding junk foods

7. Not smoking

It's never too early or too late to take the path of healthy aging. Making healthy choices can have a big impact on how you feel, both physically and mentally. You don't need to reinvent your life or lifestyle (though you may choose to down the road) but every healthy choice you make now in lieu of an unhealthy choice puts you one point further towards feeling good now, enjoying a longer life, enjoying life longer.

Chapter 2
Growing Old Obese
To grow old obese is to grow old in misery
regardless of your economic status.

It is best first to define what is meant by the terms overweight and obese. *Overweight* is defined as weighing more than the limit for your height and weight on a standard height and weight chart. *Obesity* is defined as very fat or overweight; corpulent; the condition of being obese; increased body weight caused by excessive accumulation of fat.

Historically. the most widely accepted measure of obesity has been *Body Mass Index* (BMI), calculated by dividing your weight by the square of your height. While this is no longer the primary index to obesity, it is still time honored and easy to compute. The more you weigh in relation to your height, the higher your BMI will be. You can easily calculate your own BMI:

BMI = [Weight in Pounds / (Height in inches) x (Height in inches)] x 703

A Body Mass Index of 27.3 would indicate that the person is overweight but not obese. Standard definitions are:

	BMI
Overweight	25 - 29.9
Obese	30 - 39.9
Grossly (or morbidly) obese	40+

BMI is affected by your frame size *if* you are very petite or frail, or very large boned; most of us, despite our tendency to believe that we are large boned, are medium boned. (I heard repeatedly growing up that my *bones* wouldn't fit into a size ten; obviously, they're doing okay in a four.)

BMI is also affected by your muscle mass, *if* you happen to be in excellent shape; again, most of us are not. BMI should be regarded as broadly indicative rather than as a precise measurement of health status or medical risk. You might want to calculate your own BMI now, and determine if you are overweight, obese, or morbidly obese.

I can tell you that the self acknowledgement of my own obesity came very hard for me. We can't help but admit being to being overweight or heavy, but coming to acknowledgement of our own obesity is not a pretty thing.

BMI = [Weight in Pounds / (Height in inches) x (Height in inches)] x 703

Multiply your height in inches times your height in inches, to get the square of your height.

> For example, 5'6" = 66"; 66x66=4356.

Now divide your weight by the square of your height (the number you got above from multiplying your weight by itself).

> For example: 145 divided by 4356 = 0.033.

Now multiply that result by 703.

> For Example: 0.003 x 703 = 23.1.

According to the chart, this person would be at a correct weight.

If the same person weighed 185 pounds, the BMI would be 29.8, at the high end of overweight.

At 245 the BMI is 39.5, or the high end of obese. The range referred to here as obese is known in medical offices and diet literature as *clinically obese*.

At 260 pounds, the BMI is 41.9, medically termed Grossly obese or Morbidly obese.

Your best fast check on your condition: look at your waist.

Recently, Harvard Medical School has questioned whether body mass index is a reliable method to determine whether someone is overweight. Conflicting studies, each based on BMI scores, point out flaws with the common measure, which is basically a mathematical comparison of height to weight.

New research shows that there's a better, more informative way to figure out if you are overweight: the waist-to-hip ratio.

BMI usually works well because BMI is fairly accurate when averaged across many people; but it can be way off when it comes to assessing particular individuals. It is not uncommon to get a skewed result not only for fit body builders whose BMI is high due to the extra weight associated with muscle, but also for the elderly, or those who have yo-yo dieted for many years, whose scores tend to underestimate their level of obesity because they don't take into consideration the depleted amount of muscle tissue.

The best way to determine your fat level is to measure the circumference of your waist, and then to divide that figure by the measurement of your hips.

If you're a woman, the waist-to-hip ratio should come out as no more than 0.8. Men have a little more wiggle room (no pun intended): a healthy waist-to-hip ratio for them is 0.95.

The waist-to-hip measurement is likely to catch people at risk for fat-related diseases who might think they were at a healthy weight based on their BMI score.

Just a note: we've always heard that smokers tend to gain around the middle more than others; I don't how much validity there is to this, but it is worth a thought.

As we age, many physical problems are related to the obese condition, such as difficulties in breathing, a decline in personal hygiene resulting from movement being difficult or painful, pain in the knees, and back and skin problems (which are often a direct result of Candida/Yeast overgrowth).

Obesity and its related problems may increase the risk of death at younger ages. People suffering from obesity more frequently have high blood pressure, diseases related to hardening of the arteries, blood clots in the heart and the brain, Type II (non-insulin dependent, usually brought about by obesity) diabetes, gallstones, some types of cancer, difficulties in mobility, and other conditions, maladies, and ailments. One major factor may be chronic inflammation in the body, caused by the micro flora imbalance and Yeast infestation, a state thought to contribute to illnesses such as heart disease.

Obesity is a risk factor for arthritis of the knee and hip, both potentially disabling conditions.

Recent research suggests that obesity increases chances for Alzheimer's disease/dementia. The toxins in the blood, specifically Acetaldehyde, produce many of the symptoms of a hangover: foggy brain, attention deficiency, sluggishness or fatigue, just not your usual old self. Over time, the presentation of these symptoms could even be confused medically with dementia.

Obesity directly and negatively affects the workings of our body in terms of blood volume. Blood is responsible for transportation, regulation, and protection. Blood transports nutrients and oxygen to the cells of the body, transports wastes away from cells, regulates and maintains a stable body temperature by transporting excess internal heat to the skin for evaporation, maintains our electrolyte balance and our acid/base balance, and assists in the regulation of many other body functions, including those of our hormone and immune systems.

Blood makes up about eight to ten percent of your body's weight if you are female and ten to twelve percent if you are male; the average adult has approximately two pints of blood for every twenty five pounds of body weight. So, if you weight 135 pounds (approximate average weight guideline for a female who is 5'5" tall), you are pumping about five to five and a half pints of blood through your body at all times. If you weigh 180, you're pumping more than seven pints. At 250, you pump about ten pints.

The heart pumps *all the blood in the body each minute* when the body is at rest, and every blood vessel contracts and releases with each pump, while valves work to prevent backsplash. It does not take genius to compute the workload difference on the heart and venous system at an appropriate weight to that of an overweight, obese, or morbidly obese person. Long term stress of the cardiovascular system can lead to hypertension (high blood pressure), stroke, venous and coronary disease, and heart attack. Morbidity reports repeatedly note very poor heart and vein tissue health in the obese.

Obese older adults are more likely to report symptoms of depression. These higher rates of feelings such as sadness, worthlessness, hopelessness, even despair which may be related to the social stigma, expressed both covertly and overtly, experienced by obese individuals. Negative attitudes about the obese are common, even among health care professionals and the overweight themselves. Much of the depression is a result of the toxins in the body. Feeling responsible for not being able to lose weight and the associated guilt alone can also cause depression. Negative attitudes about ourselves may be the most difficult to acknowledge at first, but they are surely present, even if unacknowledged.

Of the four top health risk factors, obesity, smoking, heavy drinking, and poverty, obesity is the most serious problem. It affects more people and is more strongly linked to very high rates of chronic illness than any of the other three risk factors.

One of the scary things as we age is the fear of falling and breaking a hip or a shoulder. Old bones do not heal quickly or easily. Being strong and keeping your reactions sharp could provide you with the ability to catch yourself in a slip or fall and possibly save you months of pain and restriction.

Recently it has been publicized that the majority of hip fractures that result from falls are actually caused by weak bones fracturing just under the weight of carrying the body, causing the fall to happen *after* the fracture occurs. Eating right to provide the nutrients required to build bone mass, and some form of exercise which causes the bone to strike a surface (such as walking), build bone tissue and can help prevent incident-free spontaneous fracturing of the hip.

Aging is something that is going to happen. It is *not* for sissies, even if you're basically healthy and fit; if you are obese, you need to start making changes now, today, and start putting into your health bank some serious care for the body you're going to get there with.

Chapter 3
The Yeast Beast Signatures: Physical and Behavioral

I believe there are several signature signs that can indicate you might have a Yeast Beast problem, particularly when multiple signs are present.

Physically, the signature is characterized by weight in the middle third of the body: large derriere, heavy thighs, 'bloating' of the stomach area. The infamous *"beer belly"* is in fact an ideal example of the bloat of the Yeast Beast; beer feeds the Beast. Heavy, hanging arms, soft thick neck, and face jowls are secondary signature signs.

People who suffer from unwanted weight gain often remark *'I just blew up"*. The weight just suddenly begins to creep on, slowly at first. Diets seem to help but then revert, often resulting in a weight higher than that when the diets were started. It is not uncommon to hear clients say they don't understand how they put on sixty-five or seventy-five pounds in eight or ten months.

Another signature is hair problems; thinning hair is the most common. Thinning hair, and losing excessive amounts of hair while brushing it or taking a shower, was my problem. I went to the doctor several times for this problem and thyroid was labeled the culprit by medical prognosis. (I had been on thyroid medication for several years; it was decided that stress and an insufficient amount of replacement thyroid was at fault. My dosage was raised. Later a follow up blood scan showed too much thyroid and my dosage was returned to the original level.) I took medicine but my hair kept falling out.

After I met Edward, while we were out walking one night (with our ankle and wrist weights) he asked me what was wrong with my hair. I was shocked, but in hindsight, I shouldn't have been, and in fact I should have made the observation myself. My hair looked really thin, dry, ragged, and just plain bad. I related my doctor stories and about a half a dozen other excuses and reasons (stress, divorce, etc.) as to why my hair was falling out and all I was doing trying to make it better. His reply to all of this was to have me order a Mason Pearson hair brush and, with three pound weights on each wrist, do 100, two handed strokes, brushing twice a day, every day. I took his advice and began this regimen.

A few months later, after I started the excess skin removal surgeries, at about the four week point I went to the hair dresser for color and style. My hairdresser remarked, "You have *a lot* of new hair growth along the scalp line; where is all the new hair coming from?" I attribute all the new growth and the ensuing improvement of the condition of my hair in general to this endeavor and the Mason Pearson brush.

* The hair loss is partly a result of the Yeast Beast, as nutrition needed for growth and healing is not received at the cellular level; Yeast steals carbon (sugar) and important amino acids, biotin (which we need to handle stress), and trace elements, none of which it can produce for its own growth. It is also a result of a sedentary lifestyle; the vigorous brushing with a quality brush (Mason Pearson is all natural boar bristle) brings the circulation, and ergo the nutrients and oxygen needed, to the follicles. Right now I'm suffering the loss of about twelve square inches of hair where it was chopped and then shaved for surgery to remove a band of excess skin from my scalp, but the rest of my hair is looking thicker and healthier than it has since I was a child.

Psychologically, orneriness, criticalness, a disagreeable and/or contrary disposition, and/or cantankerous attitude exist, particularly in the latter stages of a Candida infestation. <u>Please remember</u>: *the obese person is not likely to agree that any of this describes them*. I know *I* wouldn't have, and it took long and strong introspection after I had begun the constructive surgery phase to remove excess skin to see it. However, it is true. If you are obese, believe me: these are thing you do, too. I see this every day, as I vigilantly observe the behavior of clinically and morbidly obese people wherever I am. In fact, it still rears its ugly head on occasion, more frequently than I would like.

As you go about your

rounds, take mental fat surveys.

Next time you're at the mall, look around you: take an informal fat survey. Are the people coming towards you mostly fit or fat? We began our fat surveys in public places counting the number of people who were clinically or morbidly obese; we soon realized that the numbers of overweight, obese, and morbidly obese people in any public situation makes it easier to simply count the number of people you see who are fit and healthy looking.

Hang out around the local Starbucks; how long does it take a fit person to order, and how long does it take an obese person to order? I can tell you, though I'm a bit embarrassed about it, that, although I was unaware of the effect it had at the time, I used to create chaos at coffee places trying to get a decent Macchiato, foam on top *only* and *no* wet milk at all. *No, I said **no** wet milk in it at all; that's none, zero. Just foam on top; just floating foam on top. No wet milk period.* To me, I was nicely being assertive. Looking back, I must have been a terror to those poor young folks just trying to make a cup of coffee.

For me the process of *seeing* the people around me took months; I was completely self-trained to not see others. I didn't see what they looked like, how they looked at me, if at all, or, as I can see easily now, how people look at each other all the time. I was never aware of these things; my subconscious mind kept the information from reaching my conscious brain. I remember walking through malls when I was obese, and can honestly say that unless I saw someone grossly obese (for whom I felt sad and through whom I felt better about myself) or someone strikingly beautiful and svelte (of whom I was envious, and of whom I assumed it was a function of youth, good bones, and God's blessings) I don't remember seeing anyone at all; people just filled the mall, yet all were indistinguishable, a blur.

Later in the book I discuss the process of removing the veil from the mirror and taking– for me for the first time in over thirty years– a really honest assessment of not what *you* think you are like, but how the world reflects back to you what you really *are* like to others. This was the hardest part of my entire experience, and the most important. It is still hard for me to consciously see what the mirror is reflecting without my filters, though that's getting a little easier as I keep working on it.

Despite my photo-phobia, I utilize the still shot camera a lot. Edward will shoot forty or fifty pictures of me standing around or walking in a five or six minute period; the idea is to capture what I look like moving naturally. I am still getting used to seeing the results. Please consider utilizing the camera as you document your efforts along the way to Yeast control and weight loss. One of the things we are working on now is taking pictures of me in crowds; I truly have no mental concept of my size; I still feel fat, huge, bulky, even when the skirt tag says size 4 and it fits perfectly, even though I've been at this weight for a long time.

What people see when they ask you if you are angry (when you're not), or tell you that you seem upset or angry (when you're not) varies. The important thing is that all the synonyms for anger - rage, fury, ire, wrath, resentment, indignation - these nouns denote varying degrees of marked displeasure. Part of the anger they saw was my own self dissatisfaction; part I'm sure was job frustration. But a surprising part was that my face had gotten so large I actually had jowls, which hung down like a Sharpei's, giving me a scowling look all the time. I didn't realize this for years. Students would ask me if I was mad, and I'd be shocked. It was only when Edward told me after I had the excess skin removed from my head and neck that he had thought I had been frowning deeply all the time, and that I always appeared to look miserable and unhappy that I understood the past remarks questioning my emotional state.

According to the dictionary, the most general definition of anger is strong displeasure: *vented my anger by denouncing the supporters of the idea.* Rage and fury imply intense, explosive, often destructive emotion: *smashed the glass in a fit of rage;* directed his fury at the murderer. Ire is a term for anger most frequently encountered in literature: *"The best way to escape His ire/ Is, not to seem too happy" (*Robert Browning*).* Wrath applies especially to anger that seeks vengeance or punishment: *saw the flood as a sign of the wrath of God.* Resentment refers to indignant smoldering anger generated by a sense of grievance: *deep resentment that led to a strike.* Indignation is righteous anger at something wrongful, unjust, or evil*: "public indignation about takeovers causing people to lose their jobs"* (Allan Sloan).

I think righteous indignation most closely describes the attitude I felt most of the time. The problem is, as I look back, that righteous indignation is normally held for referring to an emotion brought about by a major wrong or miscarriage of justice; I got righteously indignant about anything I felt was wrong.

Being tired or feeling drained is also a physio-psychological signature of the Yeast Beast. This doesn't mean you can't work like a dog and out-produce others, nor does it mean you need more sleep (though you might; sleep is very important to the body's ability to heal and renew itself). What it means is that when you stop doing what you are doing for a moment you realize you are out of energy, tired, weary; this feeling often gets worse right after eating. Many cases of Chronic Fatigue Syndrome are now being attributed to Candida/Yeast infestations.

Other symptoms include insomnia, stomach ache, either constipation or diarrhea, loss of sexual desire or feeling, infertility, impotence, cold hands and/or feet, anxiety attacks, bad breath, nasal congestion, recurrent cough or bronchitis: the complete list of symptoms would take a chapter of its own. You can easily do a little searching on the WWW if you would like to know all of the symptoms attributed to Candida and other Yeast infestations.

> *More time was spent on SARS*
> *in sixty days than has been*
> *spent on Yeast in the last century.*
> *They just don't know enough*
> *about all the maladies it causes.*
> *Because of this lack of research,*
> *even __if__ the medical profession finds*
> *Yeast in various amounts, they may not*
> *know what to do with or about it.*

Yeast infections and the accompanying symptoms actually occur in stages. In the First Stage of Candida, the mucous membrane areas of the body may be infected. These include the mouth, vagina, nose, and respiratory system. You may have vaginal infections, severe P.M.S. (Pre-Menstrual Symptoms), urinary tract infections, body rashes, acne, oral thrush, jock itch, athlete's foot, allergies to foods, dust, molds, fungus, Yeast, inhalants, and chemicals; these are the most common symptoms. Repeated bouts of bronchitis, sinusitis, tonsillitis, and strep or staph infections may be typical. You may suffer bouts of mononucleosis or pneumonia. It is easy to perceive that each of these successive illnesses requires more and more antibiotics, which may open the door for further Candida overgrowth. Each instance also weakens your immune system, further providing the opportunistic little monster Yeast Beast more chances to expand.

The Second Stage of Candida may involve more generalized reactions such as pain, headaches (including migraines), extreme fatigue, psoriasis, muscle/joint aches, and arthritis. Naturally, drug after drug prescribed for symptoms is usually taken in hopes of alleviating these miserable conditions. In most cases, the symptoms alone are being treated, while the cause (Yeast overgrowth) may literally be being promoted by leveling the playing field by destroying friendly bacteria with broad spectrum antibiotics.

The Third Stage of Candida may involve mental and behavioral responses: an inability to concentrate, feeling spacey or foggy, not being able to read or follow a television program or carry on a hobby, serious forgetfulness, memory loss, mental confusion or fogginess, not being able to think of the words to say something, switching around of words and letters when trying to speak and/or write something, loss of previous skills.

These frightening problems may often lead to hopeless crying spells, severe depression, insomnia, confusion dreams, nightmares, apnea (temporary spells without breathing while sleeping), not feeling rested or restored after sleep, irrational thoughts, panic attacks, irritability, erratic behavior, violence, and even thoughts of death or suicide.

Most of these symptoms, when related to a doctor, result in diagnosis other than Yeast infestation. Sometimes people with these symptoms are labeled mentally ill, thought to be suffering from manic-depressive Psychosis or Schizophrenia. These desperately sick patients are sometimes turned over to the care of a psychiatrist or hospitalized in a mental institution. They may be given antidepressants, tranquilizers, lithium, etc. to lighten the mental symptoms, but the cause may be overlooked and the patient is not cured on a long term basis.

A person in the Fourth Stage of Candida may experience a virtual shutdown of various organ systems of the body. For example, the Digestive System may stop, producing vomiting or severe constipation. The extreme fatigue may escalate into total muscle weakness, such as the neck muscles no longer being able to hold up the head. Body rashes may escalate. The circulatory system may be swamped with so much Yeast that the capillaries become clogged, causing high blood pressure, and easy bruising.

The person may run a low-grade fever, but the hands and feet will often be very cold. The heart may develop palpitations, irregular beats, mitral valve problems or heart murmur. The alveoli (air sacs) of the lungs may be packed with Yeast so that the person cannot get adequate breath for speaking, singing, or exercise; there may be a feeling of suffocation, which may lead to hyperventilation (breathing too rapidly to get an adequate amount of oxygen) and pain. The complete failure of the Immune System leaves the body defenseless against all enemy bacteria, viruses, and disease conditions, including cancer.

The Fifth Stage of Candida seems inevitable at this point: rampant systemic Candidiasis is 100% fatal unless it is diagnosed early enough to kill the Yeast overgrowth and regenerate the Immune System.

Your awareness of these symptoms will assist you as you get the Yeast under control and lose the weight. Once treatment (Yeast control and diet) have begun, you will know within two weeks if you are on the right track.

All of my information on the maladies and conditions the Yeast Beast causes is readily available on the WWW. I found that much of the information seems unanimous, or at least readily agreed on by most, and that some of it is a little out there on the fringe. There are both lay person and scientific/medical sites available to you on line. Try doing any of the following searches, as well others, and come to your own conclusions: *Candida, Candida albicans, Yeast and Weight Loss, Candida Self Test, Yeast and Obesity, Candida Symptoms, Yeast Infestation, Yo-Yo Dieting, etc..* Again, I am not a doctor, nor do I offer this information as medical advice. Please consult with your physician or health professional.

Learn to listen to your body.

Chapter 4
Yeast and Unwilling Obesity

Yeast is a multi-specied life form from the kingdom Fungi. A normal inhabitant of the human intestines and a competitor to bacteria, Yeast population needs to be controlled and regulated. Yeast is insidious and, like many pests, once it gets a stronghold it is difficult to bring it back in line.

While in its natural state, the micro flora in our bodies is balanced and the bacteria and Yeast keep each other in check: a strong Yeast colony infestation is almost impervious to bacterial competition. Most importantly, most things we might use which are toxic to Yeast are also toxic to people.

Fungal growth takes many forms; however, Yeast is amongst the toughest and most physically protected. Also capable of mucoidal growth, a thin film-like growth is viscous (having relatively high resistance to flow; of a glutinous nature or consistency; sticky; thick; adhesive) in nature, and easily spread by natural bodily contractions: coughing, sneezing, etc. The Yeast is so small, only one to three microns in diameter, that it spreads through the body undetected and unchallenged.

It's not your fault.

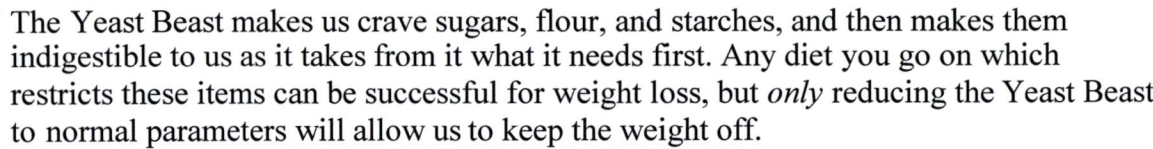

> ### *It's the Yeast Beast.*
> ### *Yeast is a biological competitor; you*
> ### *are its target, its house, and dinner.*

So many of us diet and meet with success only to regain the weight as soon as we stray from the diet. When you experience this time after time, it becomes Diet Failure Syndrome. It's not your fault, nor mine; it's the Yeast Beast.

The Yeast Beast makes us crave sugars, flour, and starches, and then makes them indigestible to us as it takes from it what it needs first. Any diet you go on which restricts these items can be successful for weight loss, but *only* reducing the Yeast Beast to normal parameters will allow us to keep the weight off.

The reason most diets fail in the long run is that most diets work in thirty to sixty days. Looking good! However, unaddressed, the overgrown Yeast Beast colony merely waits out your diet, knowing you will again soon ingest sugar, flour and starch. When you do, the Yeast Beast jumps on it right away, resulting in returned cravings, and returned weight, usually accompanied by additional weight and additional loss of overall muscle.

It takes ninety to one hundred and twenty days of diet and treatment with anti-fungals and probiotics to bring the Yeast Beast under control. How strict you are with your diet, and whether or not you decide to exercise, and how much, will strongly influence the length of time it will take you personally to get the Yeast Beast under control and lose the weight.

Please do consider taking a good multi-vitamin/mineral complex. The Yeast Beast steals from you all kinds of amino acids (crucial cellular building blocks), and biotin; these are also things your body needs for proper cell growth and repair. In addition, biotin is very important to stress control. Stress causes the body to release Cortisol, which reportedly triggers the body to store fat.

The next chapter will help you to understand the Yeast Beast.

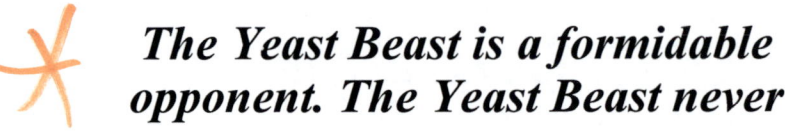

The Yeast Beast is a formidable opponent. The Yeast Beast never

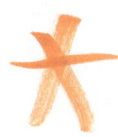

*sleeps; the Yeast Beast works on you
in your sleep. Put yourself in the
frame of mind that you are
going into a war,
a war which you will have to
win one battle at a time,
one day at a time.*

Chapter 5
Understanding the Yeast Beast
The Yeast Beast, when growing inside of you, can change
form, direction, and the object or area of infestation whenever it wants.
Get control of the Yeast Beast today, and reclaim your life.

This chapter is to help you, as a victim, friend, lover, or family member of a victim, and as a consumer, to understand the enemy, *Yeast Beast.* The Kingdom Fungi consists of mold, Yeast, rusts, smuts, mildew, and several other unnamed forms; however, for the purposes of this writing, Fungi is limited to molds and Yeast.

When first discovered, Fungi were classified a plants; later Fungi were reclassified with the status of their own kingdom. Fungi occupy many niches in our environment. However, while some of the usefulness of Fungi is a benefit to us, it should be remembered the Fungi is a biological competitor and capable of extreme prejudice. Although considered a parasite and generally non-lethal, Fungi, in particular Yeast, may infect a large percentage of our population causing conditions that affect the quality of our lives as well as our performance in life.

The Yeast Beast will make you fat, tired, sick, and a little crazy. It may make the people around you a

little crazy, too.

Fungi are an uncooperative species, and Yeast is the Trickster of the Kingdom Fungi. Bacteria, when grown in a Petri dish, make little dots of growth and stay where it is growing. Fungi, consisting of molds and Yeast, have many forms of growth (some are simply viscous and mucousy) and different growth time factors. Different Fungi may well require different culture methods and formulas to grow; they like different nutrients and different levels of pH.

Yeast and molds are not always the same after reproducing; in different environments a mold may grow as Yeast and vise versa. Many Yeast will phase, or assume different forms, when propagated for identification.

An out-of-control (overgrown) Yeast growth count means that, inside of you, Yeast is living off you and creating chemical havoc: this is the Yeast Beast. Yeast requires sugar and starch to survive and grow; it exudes toxins into your system as part of its excretion process. Just as fruit and sugar placed in a jar with household baking Yeast will ferment and create alcohol and release gas, the Yeast Beast inside you is turning your body into its own private sewer; I know this sounds gross, but it is in fact the reality.

It's all about attitude.

It is important to remember that the Yeast Beast is a life form; while not alien to this Earth or to your body, it is indeed an invading alien. It must be fought actively and vigilantly. We must declare war on this Beast. We do this by taking anti-fungals like Grapefruit Seed Extract, or Candidate (a compilation of herbs), by taking probiotics, like *Three Lac*, *Flora Five*, or *Probio 5,* by controlling our diet (very stringently at first), and, if possible, with exercise.

The whole attitude of *battling* the Yeast Beast, *being at war* with the Yeast Beast, *beating* the Yeast Beast, and *reclaiming your life* from the Yeast Beast is one you must imperatively embrace. You must realize that this truly is a "Get Out of Guilt Free Card" if you play it.

Knowing the Yeast Beast is at fault is a "Get Out of Guilt Free Card".

Play the Card. Beat The Yeast Beast.

By the way, there's a whole chapter later in the book on exercise/no-exercise; while you will undoubtedly lose weight faster, and beat the Yeast Beast faster, if you maintain a regular workout program to the level of your ability, the other weapons listed above will do the job alone if you can not or do not want to make time to exercise.

Know that exercise – even the no-exercise movements – is the nemesis of the Yeast Beast; it helps you digest your food and burn the calories; this is in direct competition to the Yeast Beasts' designs on those calories.

Chapter 6
The Fungus In Us/The Fungus On Us
Americans as a group present to the Kingdom
Fungi the grandest of opportunities for molds and Yeast.
Protected by the myopia of the health care community, this
formidable biological competitor grows in us and on us.

What is all the sudden recent attention to Yeast about? Several species of Yeast, especially *Candida albicans (C. albicans),* are becoming notorious as the source of short term, non life threatening conditions that have become medically important.

As mold inspectors, the Florida Institute of Mold has conducted numerous in-home Yeast viable (growth) surveys, and can affirmatively state that Yeast is present in most homes, and that Yeast is present in higher quantities when the inhabitants of the home are obese. Yeast is not present naturally in the outdoor environment; the Yeast we will find in your home comes from you. Part of the difficulty in Yeast control is that we continually re-ingest it throughout the day, especially in our bedrooms while we sleep.

Current spore trapping methods do not recover nor report recognizable forms of Yeast in bioaerosol cassette reports of Fungi by laboratories analyzing bioaerosol cassettes. While it is perhaps not appropriate to go into all the scientific reasons for this*, the bottom line is that in thousands upon thousands of bioaerosol cassettes taken in homes around the county, many molds are recovered, but Yeast is never reported; they just do not know how to recover it. I believe Florida Institute of Mold, and its Multi-Species Optimum Recovery Laboratory may currently be the *only* multi-species Yeast optimum recovery laboratory in the nation.

*If you are interested in the reasons why Yeast is not ever recovered in the analyzing of bio-aerosol cassette reports of Fungi by laboratories you can check our website, floridainstituteofYeast.com/Challenge.html)

Yeast is a natural inhabitant of your body which only becomes a threat when it is allowed the opportunity to grow out of control.

Yeast in our bodies is usually commensal (of, relating to, or characterized by a symbiotic relationship in which one species is benefited while the other is unaffected). Multi-antibiotic treatment may be the start of a virulent Yeast Candida growth as may many other factors. Unfortunately, the Yeast count in *your* body is *your* Yeast count and Yeast counts vary from person to person.

As there is no benchmark for an acceptable Yeast count in the human body, the only way to know what is going on is to test yourself on an on going basis. Real Yeast testing which will recover a broad spectrum of Yeast is not without cost; it is easier and less expensive to presume an out of control level of Yeast and consult your physician or health care professional.

Self diagnosis and treatment are growing in popularity. Florida Institute of Mold offers the Candida Self Test as a tool for self diagnosis. The Candida Self Test has not been reviewed or approved by the FDA or any recognized medical body. It will recover Yeast and mold from expelled saliva, skin surfaces, and skin folds. The Candida Self Test is not meant to replace your doctor's advice; please consult your doctor or licensed health care professional for medical advice. (If you are interested, please see our websites, floridainstituteofmold.com or floridainstituteofyeast.com. There is a coupon at the back of this book for a discount on a Personal Yeast Test Kit if you are would like to pursue self testing.)

You disperse Yeast in your home, car, and office. This is correct; the major source of Yeast in the air of your home is you, your family, and your pets. Usually found in the bedroom, bathroom, and kitchen, Yeast is difficult to spore trap and difficult to recover (grow). It takes Yeast up to three weeks to mature for identification.

Yeast testing is not without cost, and is not necessary unless you want to know what Yeast is growing on and in you. If you are over fifty pounds overweight, you have Yeast problems, and you, your family, and pets are ingesting the Yeast in their sleep. My suggestion is that you assume you do have Yeast, and get yourself and your family and house pets on anti-fungals (I'd begin with Grapefruit Seed Extract) and probiotics (I'd begin with Three Lac.)

These and other helpful supplements can be purchased on most of our websites: beautyandtheyeastbeast.com, ijustblewup.com, or endtheobesity.com. (There is a complete list of our websites and several discount coupons at the end of the book.) These products can also be ordered elsewhere on the web, and some are available in health food stores. It doesn't matter where you get the supplements that will help you start recovering soon: just get started on them *as soon as possible.*

Chapter 7
On Fungal Detection and Identification
Understudied, uncooperative, tricky and just plain ornery: with Fungi, more often than not, the exception is the rule.

In the laboratory world of microbiology, getting bacteria samples identified is fairly easy. Many laboratories now specialize in the identification of molds by spore identification (non viable) and or growth (viable) identification. When querying laboratories about Yeast identification, very few will identify Yeast to the genus level if they can identify it at all. There are no Yeast propagating laboratories I know of besides Florida Institute of Mold.

What I have found, as a mold inspector and the owner of a licensed fungal micro propagation laboratory (Florida Institute of Mold's Optimum Recovery Laboratory optimumrecoverylabs.com), is that conventional laboratory methods are inadequate and antiquated for the multi-species optimum recovery of molds and Yeast for identification. (Again, if you have interest in this specifically, you can check our website, floridainstituteofYeast.com/Challenge.html.)

Doctors are usually interested in a particular organism, such as *Candida albicans*; therefore the laboratory cultures the specimens specifically for *Candida albicans*. This is known as a *single species recovery*. If there other Yeast or molds present, they are suppressed or inhibited from growth chemically in the process of micro propagation (growth) by altering the agar, or growing media.

Laboratories which identify molds by growth, or viable mold, testing generally use a single agar Petri dish to recover molds and Yeast from samples. Single plate recovery culture is unacceptable as a method to recover molds and Yeast if identifying all the molds and Yeast in a sample is important.

As a victim of the Yeast Beast, I certainly would have liked to have known how much of what kind of Yeast was growing inside of me! I currently test myself and others regularly for the presence and count of Yeast and I can definitely assure you that there is a lot more than Candida albicans growing in most of us. We carry a number of different Yeast, as well as numerous molds.

I should note here that self testing is <u>not</u> required. If you are more than fifty pounds overweight, you can just *assume* you have a Yeast infestation and begin a recovery program. I test myself monthly just to keep an eye on how much Yeast is showing up just so I have a sense of normal for my body and therefore some warning when the number of colonies in a sample starts climbing. I have a number of clients who also want this information; some of them actually utilize the test results to modify their diet and exercise; some just want to know.

These are my concerns as a Yeast sufferer and a licensed Obesity Counselor. However, as a Certified Mold Inspector and the owner of a fungal micro propagation laboratory, I want to know *all* the molds and Yeast in a sample. I culture all samples, environmental and personal, for all molds and Yeasts. This type of culture is referred to as *multi-species optimum recovery.*

Fungal infestation in single family dwellings and office buildings is currently causing great dispute as to how sick fungus can make you. The debate goes on about the effects of Fungi on our health. There is now dialog on the environment as a source of fungal infestation in the human body, both as allergens and pathogens, causing human illness. Doctors are now prescribing anti-fungals for acne, rather than antibiotics. While there are still many doctors out there who think Candida is a hoax, the numbers are shrinking every year. Many doctors now prescribe anti fungals at the same time they prescribe antibiotics to avoid opportunistic Yeast overgrowth.

Nail fungus, jock itch, vaginal itch, eczemas, and a myriad of other ailments are the result of fungus. It is only recently that the health and medical professions are looking here for answers; more research was done on SARS in sixty days than has been done on Fungi in the last century.

One important thing to realize about

Obesity is that it is the
fungal infestation you can see.

Chapter 8
Guilt: Yours, Mine, Our Families' and Friends'
*Guilt over unexplained weight gain and non-understandable diet
failure brings about very strained emotions and relationships.*

The Yeast Beast, the Yeast Syndrome: however you term it, the out-of-control Yeast population that causes uncontrolled overweight issues often leads to yo-yo dieting, and finally to Diet Failure Syndrome and unwilling morbid obesity.

Diet Failure Syndrome: repeated post-diet return of weight, usually with additional weight gain and loss of muscle tissue, despite the original level of success of the diet.

The fact is that as you lose the weight, you *must* starve the Yeast Beast to be successful, and, once starved and kept dormant, *then* – and only then – can you take over control of your weight and successfully bring it within normal bounds and keep it there with any longevity.

The problem with most diets is that people go on them for about sixty days. It takes

39

ninety to one hundred and twenty days of dieting, *and* taking anti-fungals and probiotics, to beat the Yeast Beast back to normal levels. When we diet alone, the weight usually comes back on as soon as we end a diet or move to a maintenance plan and start adding foods which promote the Yeast Beast again, because the actual cause of the weight gain, the Yeast Beast, was never addressed or remedied.

How much guilt can one carry about being overweight? Growing up fat with a sister who was a size five/seven (down to a three after giving birth to my niece) wasn't much fun. I was haunted for years by a brief shopping trip with her after the birth of my niece, where she cried to me because they didn't have anything smaller than a 4/5 while at the same time I was unable to find anything to find anything because they didn't have anything bigger than an 18/20. I was 16 years old.) Having two brothers, one overweight, but a jock, and one thin and delicate boned, I certainly felt that Someone Upstairs had sent the wrong bodies down for at least two of us. But I was the only one who was obese.

How could I not think it my fault, my lack of willpower, my shortcoming? How could anyone around me not think those things of me? In fact, I was accused of those things upon many occasions. Telling a person who has a Yeast infestation to lose weight and not helping them to get the infestation under control is a lot like telling an alcoholic to stop drinking without giving them any help to get the alcoholism under control. There are alcoholics who successfully remain dry for periods of time; however, unless the alcoholism is addressed, these efforts are destined to fail.

How can we diet and lose but always regain and it *not* be our/their fault? If you are considerably overweight or obese, or you have a sibling, spouse, friend, lover or other you care about who is obese, this may be the most important fact in this book:

*It is **<u>not</u>** your fault.*
*It is not **<u>their</u>** fault.*
It is the Yeast Beast.

Chapter 9
For Victims, Families, and Friends
Unwilling obesity, unwanted, misunderstood, and the cause of tremendous
tension and strain in relationships: one of the objectives of this book is
to tell everybody: you're off the hook for guilt.

I believe that unwilling obesity in Americans is caused by an imbalance in the micro flora of a person's body that favors the growth of Yeast. This Yeast imbalance causes not only unwilling obesity: medical experts site a myriad of other conditions and illnesses caused by Yeast imbalance.

The mystery of the diet yo-yo syndrome that, until the printing of this book, has been misunderstood and unexplainable is now solved; it is **The Yeast Beast** that is the cause. Everyone involved in this family tragedy of unwilling obesity can now face the problem realizing that *everyone* is a victim: the obese person, his/her parents, siblings and other relatives, friends, lovers, and spouses. I don't know what frustration or embarrassment I caused my family over the years regarding my weight, but I know that the difficulties in my personality, which started as a teen and got worse until I was fifty-five, created years of strain and stress on my relationships with my parents, siblings, daughter and grandchildren, as well as my previous husband.

Earlier in the book I mentioned blowing up when I was five. I was one of four children in the family; my mother doesn't remember specific details of minor childhood incidents, but, as I had chronic tonsillitis, bronchitis, and/or strep every year of my life as far back as I *can* remember until I had my tonsils taken out at eighteen, it is my belief that even before I was old enough to remember, I had probably been given broad spectrum antibiotics at least once, and probably several times.

Antibiotics, and especially broad spectrum antibiotics, kill off large numbers of bad bacteria, which is wonderful. Unfortunately, they also kill off large numbers of beneficial, friendly bacteria; this leaves the playing field open for the Fungi, and Fungi are opportunistic little Beasts which never miss the chance to increase their territory. Once the balance is disturbed, and the Fungi spread, their toxins begin to affect you, and the major symptom is weight gain.

Uncontrolled weight gain overall, in spite of periodic losses, can lead to several other complications; however, the psychological factor is the first issue that needs to be addressed by the victim and the victim's family and friends. The psychological factor is two pronged: part of it is the anger and frustration caused by repeated failure, and part of it is the second and third stage effects of Yeast on the body and the psyche, which *cause* anger and frustration as well as a critical, obstinate, contentious, or ornery attitude.

Keep in mind that any discussion of anger/frustration/ornery behavior requires that the overweight, obese, or morbidly obese person be able to identify that there is a pervasive presence of these attitudes; I never felt angry (as a pervasive attitude) but I can see clearly now in how many sneaky ways anger reared its ugly, denied, insidious, unconscious self. Even now, I fight old patterns, ever watchful for slips of passive-aggressive behavior, creating chaos, and other self-focusing activities I swear to you I would have denied to the death ever having or ever exhibiting prior to having come to terms with the Curse of the Yeast Beast; I freely admit that there are still times where it gets the best of me and I can't see it until after it's happened.

If you love or live with an obese person, you can probably assume that they have Yeast. If they have been overweight for a long time, you can assume that they are into one of the latter stages of Yeast Infestation. By the way, if you have lived with an overweight person for some time, you may want to check your own Yeast levels; the Yeast expelled and released by the body of an obese person is inhaled by others, including pets, in the house.

The Yeast Beast can make you
cranky, ornery, disagreeable,
nit-picky, cantankerous, contentious…
just a <u>little</u> hard to live with.

And – it can come and go,
making the person you live
with or love think you are bi-polar at times.

Chapter 10
I Know My Lies, Your Lies, Our Lies
***This is a tough chapter. It was difficult in my life, it is difficult in the
writing, and it is probably difficult in your life. Be brave; have courage;
the truth only hurts the first time. (Well, the first is the worst.)***

I spent forty years overweight and obese to the point of unwilling morbid obesity
(defined as one hundred or more pounds overweight). It is with great difficulty that I
write this chapter because, even as I am in the final phase of my metamorphosis, I have
discovered that the self deceptions one lives with can, over time, create a reality that is
based on self deceit; it is a delusional reality.

"Mirror, Mirror, on the wall:
Who's the fairest of them all?"
The Wicked Queen, <u>Snow White</u>

What do you *see* when you look in the mirror? Truthfully: do you *look*? The mirror can
be a very friendly or very *un*friendly thing; when the mirror is unfriendly for a long,
long time, you tend to stop consciously acknowledging the image before you. I know I
did. And your mind hides from you the fact that you are not consciously receiving the
image, so you aren't even aware you see but don't see.

Every morning when I woke up I was disappointed, discouraged, dissatisfied with my life; I was not aware of this of course; it has been blocked from consciousness as has the image in the mirror, which we learn to see, but not see. I begin the day choosing something to wear. Now, at 250-300 pounds, the truth is nothing really looks well or attractive no matter how lovely the fabric, design, or style is, and all I am doing is trying to look appropriate and, more importantly, trying to hide the fat. I am in fact hiding from the reality of it all, and from the fact that when you are obese some things may look better than others, but nothing makes you look not obese. But while I know, of course, that I am overweight, I do not concede to myself that I am obese. I am not aware of the myriad of other distortions and illusions in my reality. My reality becomes delusional in many ways.

As I face the world, I know people will look beyond the weight and see me for my better qualities. ***Oh, really?*** I can tell you one thing for sure: I always believed this and never had any idea this was a false premise until after I faced the past with the veil down. This is going to hurt, folks: people see fat people as fat, as lazy, as having no self control, as having little self-respect, as being less productive, as being a health insurance risk, as…. Need I go on?

But *"This looks okay"*, as if putting the outfit made me look okay as in *'not fat'*, is the underline unacknowledged lie that started my day every day. My husband at the time was a good man and a kind person, and told me *every morning* I looked good, great, beautiful, special that day. He never would have thought doing so was assisting me in maintaining a delusional picture of myself and my life. I never believed I ever looked as good as he always said I did, but I must have not looked that bad if he was repeatedly generous with compliments, so I accepted his generous compliments as solid feedback that I looked okay and, since my image of myself was based on mental creation only, I used this false feedback to confirm my false reality.

Had I ever been able to stand in front of the mirror full body naked and *actually let in the reflection being shown to me come through to awareness,* I would have known his compliments were coming from his not wanting to hurt me, from loving me and wanting me to have a good day, but not from a truthful reaction to what he saw.

***When you look at an obese person,
you unconsciously assume that
s/he sees what you see. The
majority of obese people consider***

*themselves overweight, not obese, even
at 200+ on the scale. Most are shocked when
they see a picture of themselves, which
freezes one glance and makes the true
body image static and real. Most fat people
hate photographs of themselves. Lots
of us become the family picture
takers, hiding behind the camera.*

When, as a parent, spouse, friend or lover, you are dealing with an individual with an uncontrolled weight problem, and you do not realize or understand the cause of the gain is a Yeast problem, it seems that there is no reasonable answer. If there is no reasonable answer, reason leaves.

Many of us have the experience of cutting back our calories severely, only to find that the body takes this new caloric limit and *lowers* the body's metabolism to survive on it, making it harder to lose weight and creating a situation where eating a normal amount of calories causes weight gain.

To the victim, the Yeast infestation causing insane cravings and weight gain on very small volumes of food is an inexplicable phantom, a specter which leaves unconscious and/or unacknowledged self-doubt and anger. It is only sane for most people to assume that everyone is responsible for what they eat and what they weigh. *If I have a problem with my weight it's a result of my lack of will power and fortitude; there must be something wrong with me.*

Yo-yo dieting only increases and reinforces this self-doubt. *Why does every diet I try start off okay and then things go right back where they were? What is <u>wrong</u> with me?* Still needing to function in the world, self-deceptions by means of blocking consciousness and telling unconscious or semi-conscious little white lies to ourselves become the mitigator of insanity.

When my niece was little, she would say, "*Mirror, mirror on the wall, who's the fetchit of them all.*" At the time, it was just cute; it was a nonsense word. But in retrospect, it becomes an interesting linguistic play. *Fetchit,* while not a real word, is summarily what I made of my life; fetch it at work, fetch it for a man, fetch it for acceptance; it was never that I was trying to buy attention or affection, but my self esteem was low despite many accomplishments in my life, and I believe I bent and twisted myself to fit in places where I just never felt like I fit. Much of my own personality shifted and warped over the years, ever seeking to fit the square peg of me into the round world.

One of the hardest things I work on today is trying to get my self-image to coincide with the image the rest of the world receives, both in regards to my physical presence and my psychological one.

Chapter 11
Eating for Two
The Yeast Beast is a master of chemistry and yours has
been made openly available with no contest. The Yeast Beast
has been controlling your eating habits through chemistry.

Most women understand the phrase, *eating for two*; it usually means whomever is being referred to is pregnant. When we refer to *eating for* two in this book, we mean eating for you and the Yeast Beast.

Are you living with an addict?

The Yeast Beast is a sugar addict, a flour addict, a potatoes and pasta and cake and rice and noodles and pie and Danish and bagel addict. The Yeast Beast craves these things for its survival. Unlike unfriendly bacteria, which seek to harm you and make you ill, Yeast Beast is interested in your survival. In fact, it's interested in your survival *and* your continued size expansion; a bigger you is a bigger Yeast Beast home.

One of the problems with eating to calm the Yeast Beast is that you ingest foods that are high in glycemic index – high in the sugars and starches that go right to the hips, tummy, and tush.

Compounding the problem is that the Yeast Beast steals what it needs from the sugar and starch and leaves you with fairly indigestible food, the stuff that gives you constipation, gas, bloating, and toxins floating around your system. High glycemic foods (high sugar/starch) provide Yeast with the Carbon it needs. Yeast also steals from you important amino acids and other minerals, trace elements, and biotin, things which it needs to reproduce and grow but cannot itself produce; they are all things your body needs to work effectively.

Women who have been pregnant often swear the *baby* is craving ice cream, or pizza, or Twinkies; whatever the need, and while it is true that the body will crave what it (or its embryo) needs, these sugar and starch cravings are coming from the Yeast Beast, not the Body. The body makes you crave things like orange juice or lemonade when you are low on vitamin C, or steak and eggs when you're low on protein. The Yeast Beast craves sugar and flour: cookies, candies, cake, bread, pasta, pancakes; the favorite fix usually combines all three Yeast Beast essentials: sugar, flour and fat.

We need to learn to listen to our bodies, and hear what they are asking for. (Many of us need to learn to hear the body's request for water, not food; it is a request often misinterpreted.) And we need to learn to recognize which voice is talking, Body or Beast. Like a multiple personality, both claim ownership of you, and both make their demands accordingly, neither caring much about the needs of the other.

The easiest way to hush the Yeast Beast, which also makes it a lot easier to hear your body when it talks to you, is to remove all sources of sugar, flours, and starches. The Yeast Beast will scream at first (see Chapter 17, Supplements, for an explanation of *Beast Burn Off*), but it grows quiet after about three days on Phase One of the diet.

If you have any concerns at all about changing your diet quickly, you can give yourself an extra week of a pre-Phase One, where you add to the restrictive diet enough fruit and perhaps a small portion of cereal or rice to being staving off the Yeast Beast, but not throwing it, or your body, into discomfort; this will make the first week on the straight diet easier for you. If you do a pre-Phase One week, do not take the anti fungals for that week, but do begin taking the probiotics.

The war with the Yeast Beast is won one battle at a time.

Once you begin battling the Yeast Beast, after the initial three or four days, you will find that you no longer eat for two; you eat for your health and well being, and to keep the

Yeast Beast at bay. The cravings you have lived with for bread and sugar and the like will diminish; in fact, the longer you stay on the Phase One program the less your desire becomes even after the initial decrease. You will notice that you choose to eat only when you're hungry after a few days, and that you will eat what you need and stop most of the time. Do make sure you are eating frequently and getting enough protein. When you are on an all protein with salad diet, you need to keep the body revved up with protein through the day; somehow, it's part of how the chemistry of the body works under protein to burn fat.

As you complete the first week and move into the second, you will find that as you do so, your energy improves, your focus and clarity improve, your skin may improve, your weight goes down, and your attitude goes up. Actually, it *is* a little like being pregnant!

Chapter 12
Overweight Weak/Overweight Strong

Many of the overweight population in this country have never been strong. Being strong means you should be able to sustain thirty minutes of vigorous physical activity which utilizes both your upper and lower body.

As a nation we are informational giants: mechanically enhanced, but physically weak. Most scary to me, we are raising a generation of obese children. Childhood obesity has been in the news in increasing amounts. Having been an obese child, I know what that is like; I know what the future holds if it is not resolved, and I know what old age will present if the obese condition is allowed to persist.

Most fit people are at an appropriate weight for their height and age. Some fit people are too thin, but they are still fit. Some are too heavy, but they are still fit. To be seriously overweight and still be strong, one would have to be a body builder or serious sports participant. Many heavy men seem strong because they were at one time athletic and they know how to use their weight to move things; few of the men who can move a dresser across the room for you with ease could pick up and carry that same dresser around the house for a half hour.

My husband has a measure of fitness that is easy to test: sitting in a sturdy armed chair, grasp the arms and push yourself up, holding your legs out in front of you, parallel to the seat of the chair: if you can lift and hold yourself off the chair in that position for sixty seconds, you're not in bad a shape in relation to your weight. (Please don't misunderstand: this is not the acid test for what is strong. Many strong and fit people cannot do this. But if you *can* do it, you're strong.

Nothing makes old age harder than immobility.

Women are especially under muscled, both because of genetics and mostly non-physical labor vocations; this is defiantly detrimental to our health, especially as we age. You must be strong and supple to catch yourself and prevent or to recover from a slip. If you are overweight, and you are not fit, you are probably going to go down if you slip. If you are not supple and you slip and fall you could easily break something, such as your hip or your shoulder; both of these are painful and long healing injuries, often requiring surgery to place pins in the bone, and repeat surgery to remove them. Getting strong and supple is a requirement of obesity recovery and an important part of avoiding advanced infirmation (see Chapter 2).

This program promises a 'no-exercise' option for those that want it; I did lose the first 125 pounds without exercise. But remember, you are looking to make yourself fit to live in old age. Nothing makes old age harder than immobility. You must begin to awaken your muscles and plan to start doing exercise and building them up later.

To get your energy level up, take your anti fungals and begin a program to get moving. Remember, if you are obese *any* sustained movement will be at first difficult. There are pictures later in the book of non-strenuous, muscle awakening moves you can do in front of the TV: wave your arms side to side slowly, lift your feet and set them down again, etc. Walk when you can. Park just a little further away from the store. Try walking *down* the stairs even if you used the elevator to go up.

Begin doing hand and foot movements with weights; we suggest wearing low weight (one pound on each hand and foot to start) just while going through your normal day, or at least around the house. Turn on some music; you may not have the energy to dance right now, but you can begin to sway with the music, bend your knees a little, and move your arms in the air. Muscles respond to music and actually have music memory. Introduce your muscles now to music you can work out to later as you progress. We make our own CD's on the computer to control the type of music we like, the length of the songs (we alternate long and short songs to increase efficiency of our workouts), and the variation of tempo in the songs (working out alternating slow and fast pace maximizes the workout).

If you want to live longer and not suffer advanced infirmation you just need to get moving: go dancing, walking with weights, do arm exercises while sitting; do anything but just get moving. The faster your metabolism is working the harder you are fighting the Yeast Beast. The faster your metabolism is working, the faster your body will burn excess fat. A higher metabolism will also flush toxins and poisons which have been stewing inside of you for a long time. You will find that drinking a lot of water will assist your body in releasing these toxins.

When you are obese and sedentary, you are creating a later life scenario of health problems and a shortened life span.

If you are obese you need to understand that you have become an enslaved source for what the Yeast Beast wants, and how it goes about getting you to procure it for him, all at great cost to you. Take your life back; work the Yeast Beast out of you.

Chapter 13
Sick Structure Syndrome

In the mold industry we talk of Sick Building Syndrome when a building is infested with molds. When any structure gets sick with mold, be it an apartment complex, a condo, a house, a school or an office building, the term Sick Building Syndrome describes a situation in which reported symptoms among a population of building occupants can be temporally associated with their presence in that building as a result of something in the air which is effecting them. This something is very often mold.

The symptoms of Sick Building Syndrome include common maladies such as headaches, respiratory infections, asthma, and serious allergies. Additional symptoms related to Sick Building Syndrome include cough, chest tightness, fever, chills, muscle aches, and allergic reactions such as mucous membrane irritation and upper respiratory congestion.

Generally, a wide spectrum of complaints is involved. Additional complaints may include an inability to concentrate, and general malaise-complaints suggestive of a host of common ailments, some ubiquitous and easily communicable. The key factors are commonality of symptoms amongst the inhabitants or workers of the building (or home) and the absence of these symptoms among building occupants when the individuals are not in the building.

Sick building syndrome should be suspected when a substantial proportion of those spending extended time in a building (as in daily employment or as in the home) report or experience acute on-site discomfort. If you go away for the weekend, and while you're gone you awaken feeling better, more refreshed, and less stuffy, and if you sleep better while away than you do at home, your home is a sick structure, and is likely highly contaminated with molds and Yeast or both.

Houses, condos, apartments, offices, commercial units: these are all different kinds of buildings, different kinds of structures. Your body is also a structure. When you are infested with high Yeast counts, the same thing happens to your body as to any building structure: the inhabitant/occupant (you) gets ill. We use the term Sick *Structure* Syndrome to include the list of problems and ailments that affect any structure, whether brick and mortar or cells and tissues.

Your body is both house and host to Fungi (Yeast and molds). In an uninfested body, there is a delicate balance between good/friendly bacteria and Fungi. This balance between the friendly bacteria and the Fungi is the key to maintaining good health. When the balance is disrupted and the bacteria prevail, we get sick: fever, infection, etc. When the imbalance allows the Yeast to prevail, we get generally unwell, and many kinds of illness may follow, but we don't get necessarily sick with fevers and infections and life threatening diseases. Bacteria can threaten your life; the Yeast Beast threatens your *quality* of life. Do note, however, that, left untreated, if the infestation moves into the later stages, your very life could indeed be threatened by the damage being done to your organs by the rampaging colonies.

If you have never taken steps to combat the Yeast inside of you and you are overweight, you can appropriately assume that you do have excessive Yeast. This Yeast condition will not change without a fight. Yeast is an organism that wants to live and grow big and make lots of more Yeast. Bacteria may want to hurt you, but the Yeast Beast wants you alive and well and creating more territory for it to live in.

Sick Structure Syndrome in your home or sick Structure Syndrome of the body; they go hand in hand. I have mentioned, the Yeast in our homes primarily comes from us. When we are infested with Yeast we exude it in our breath, our sweat, and our shedding skin cells.

If you culture droplets of rain as they fall, you will find a myriad of molds but no Yeast; Yeast is not normally present in an outdoor environment. Yeast is found in homes where people are. Some comes from our cooking, but most Yeast in the home comes from the bodies of the human residents, and the majority of Yeast in the home is found in the bedroom and bathrooms, where it is shed as we shower, change, and sleep.

*You can live with termites for years
and not know you have them until
your house starts crumbling; the Yeast Beast
operates in the same insidious manner.*

Sick Structure Syndrome – Sick Body Syndrome – either way, it is imperative to identify the situation and take steps to remedy it. An untreated structure, building or body, will only continue to get sicker and eventually need condemnation (hospitalization) if ignored.

Chapter 14
The Diet

When I was yo-yo dieting over a period of some thirty years, I met with small, moderate, and great successes on various diets; of course, none of them ever failed to leave me climbing back up the scale, usually to new heights. This is because I never took on the Yeast Beast.

This is not a diet book; this is a guide to controlling Yeast infestation, which will then allow you to achieve permanent weight loss. It includes a diet to help starve off the Yeast Beast. The entire package is one of naturopathy; naturopathy incorporates a variety of natural approaches (actively through diet, nutrition, supplements, and exercise, and passively through rest, deep breathing, and relaxation) to promote health and well-being on all levels: body, mind and spirit.

Doing the regimen required to battle the Yeast Beast – the anti-fungals, the probiotics, and the immune system enhancers – is half the job; diet and exercise (or no-exercise) and deep breathing, rest, and relaxation compose the other half.

If you're like me, you're already wondering why it took this far into the book to get to the diet (and if you're *really* like me, you've already scoped the table of contents and come here first), and now you're thinking you have to read through the naturotherapy stuff now, too; happily, the rest of this chapter focuses on the diet, and the supplements, exercise (or no-exercise), deep breathing, rest, and relaxation are covered in future chapters.

The truth about diets: folks, *ALL* diets work. Everyone's body is different, and whether you believe in diet by blood type, body shape, astrological sign, ethnic background, or any number of other diet type descriptor programs that are out there or not, different diets work differently for different people. Different body needs (protein, carb, fat types) and different tastes and cultural biases, different work schedules and family situations: these things all contribute to the levels at which different diets are palatable for different people, and also partially determine how successful each diet can be for different individuals.

I am sure you could tell me right now how many diets you've been on in your life, and how each worked for you, or not, and which were the easiest for you to follow, and which brought you the most success.

Here is the very best news: once you declare war on the Yeast Beast, get the regimen up to battle level, and complete the initial four week siege (starve back) against the Yeast Beast, *you can move to any diet you ever liked and had success on and lose all the weight your body needs to lose.*

My body happens to be highly carbohydrate intolerant, and I have food allergies to sugar, flour, corn, soy, and chocolate, so, while I do eat these foods now, I do so in limited amounts and listen to my body vigilantly. I also step up my workout when I know I'm eating more of these things. When I was losing the weight, I stayed on the second phase of the diet for several years, allowing myself 'cheats' along the way after losing the first fifty pounds. Cheats are always taken one cheat at one sitting and never with frequency while you are still losing weight. My favorite cheat was cheesecake; if I left the crust off, I was actually staying within the diet framework except for the sugar in the body of the cheese cake. (I'd take the white top off if it had one, too; the topping has more sugar than the rest of the piece of cake!) We'll also talk later about exercise 'legalizing' cheating.

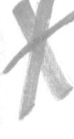Candida and other Yeast infestations can be controlled by means of the elimination of certain foods in order to create an acidic internal environment deplete of Carbon(sugar and starch) sources in which the Yeast cannot thrive, coupled with the anti-fungal, probiotics, and immune system supplements, which ensure that the levels of systemic Candida are significantly reduced. Thereafter, a maintenance program should be followed to keep your micro flora balanced. We will discuss maintenance and self-testing options later.

Remember that Candida and other Yeast thrive on *all sugars, complex and refined carbohydrates* and it is only by controlling your intake of these foods that you will beat systemic Candida or other Yeast. By following this diet, you will not only be able to control Yeast levels in your body, but you will also be amazed at the ease with which you are able to lose weight, despite the fact that on Phase One there are no limitations to the amounts you can eat, only the choices available.

By reducing the Candida (or other Yeast) overgrowth in the body, the immune system is able to function and heal properly for the first time in years; as a result, many people report clearer skin, a reduction of joint or muscle pain, a balancing of sugar levels and/or blood pressure, cholesterol coming under control, relief from symptoms of depression, and a myriad of other 'miracles' that happen as a result of the diet and the successful Yeast Beast battle.

This point is paramount, and bears repeating:

> ***You may not use sugar in <u>any</u> form; this includes glucose, sucrose (cane sugar), and fructose (fruit sugar). Lactose (milk sugar) must be kept to a minimum; the higher the fat content of the milk, the lower the sugar content.***

We never use anything lighter than half and half, and we use whole milk yogurt and real butter (lots of butter).

The Diet

Foods To Avoid Throughout *ALL* Phases

Anything containing Yeast
Any kind of sugar (anything ending in –ose is a sugar)
Pickled, smoked, or processed meat
Ketchup
Breads, rolls, cakes, etc.
All flour, semolina, pasta

Cream of wheat
All vinegars and vinegar products
Salad dressings
Processed cheeses (American cheese, cheese spreads)
Grapes
Any fruit or vegetable showing any signs of bruising or mold
All fruit juices
All dried fruits
Honey and other natural sweeteners
Artificial sweeteners
All forms of alcohol (alcohol is a form of sugar)

Phase One – Two Weeks

Unlimited quantities of protein:
> Poultry (chicken, turkey, game hens)
> Fish/Shellfish (all types allowed)
> Salmon (particularly beneficial)
> Meat (beef, pork, lamb, buffalo)
> Cheese (best are Jack, Mozzarella, cream cheese; cheddars, Brie, and
>> various semi-soft cheeses have lower effectiveness on the Yeast Beast
>> control as well as the weight loss)
> Eggs

Unlimited quantities of salad greens only: Lettuce (all the fun kinds, but not
> Iceberg), raw spinach, raw cabbage

Butter, olive oil and garlic as desired

Seasonings which contain no sugars or artificial sweeteners (remember, anything that
> ends in –ose is a sugar)

Lemon juice (up to two tablespoons a day)

Black/unsweetened coffee, tea, bottled waters and sparkling waters

Phase Two – Two Weeks

Unlimited quantities of protein:
> Poultry (chicken, turkey, game hens)
> Fish/Shellfish (all types allowed)
> Salmon is particularly beneficial
> Meat (beef, pork, lamb, buffalo)
> Cheese (best are Jack, Mozzarella, cream cheese; cheddars, Brie, and

various semi-soft cheeses have lower effectiveness on the Yeast Beast control as well as the weight loss)

       Eggs

Easy Greens (this refers to the very low carbohydrate, mostly green, vegetables): Lettuce (all the fun kinds, but not Iceberg), broccoli, cauliflower, spinach, cabbage, cucumbers, bell peppers (preferably red, yellow and orange), asparagus, leek, onion, etc.

Butter, olive oil and garlic as desired

Seasonings which contain no sugars or artificial sweeteners (remember, anything that ends in –ose is a sugar.)

Lemon juice (up to two tablespoons a day)

Black/unsweetened coffee, tea, bottled waters and sparkling waters

Phase Three Two Weeks

Unlimited quantities of protein:
       Poultry (chicken, turkey, game hens)
       Fish/Shellfish (all types allowed) Salmon is particularly beneficial
       Meat (beef, pork, lamb, buffalo)
       Cheese (best are Jack, Mozzarella, cream cheese; cheddars, Brie, and various semi-soft cheeses have lower effectiveness on the Yeast Beast control as well as the weight loss)
       Eggs

Easy Greens (this refers to the very low carbohydrate, mostly green, vegetables): Lettuce (all the fun kinds, but not Iceberg), broccoli, cauliflower, spinach, cabbage, cucumbers, bell peppers (preferably red, yellow and orange), asparagus, leek, onion, etc.

Butter, olive oil and garlic as desired

Seasonings which contain no sugars or artificial sweeteners (remember, anything that ends in –ose is a sugar.)

Lemon juice (up to two tablespoons a day)

Black/unsweetened coffee, tea, bottled waters and sparkling waters

In this phase you can add one *fruit a day* in week one. (Berries are best, or apple; NO grapes, and never any dried or bruised fruit. Tomatoes are actually fruits, and you may have a fresh tomato as a fruit.) It is suggested you watch how you feel, how your clothing fits, and the scale, and adjust accordingly. I am particularly carbohydrate sensitive, and chose to only eat ½ cup of berries or one small apple every few days when I am on my periodic Yeast Maintenance Yeast Beast starve-backs.

In week two, after you are okay with your response to fruit, you can also add a source of grain twice a week: ½ cup of oatmeal (no sugar or milk), or ½ cup of brown rice, or two Rye Crisp crackers, or one piece of rye bread (Rye bread and crackers contain no Yeast), or two brown rice cakes, or ½ avocado.

In this phase you can now also add one cup of plain unflavored whole milk yogurt. You may have one on any day you are not having grain. You can sweeten it with your ½ cup of berries or other fruit if you don't like the taste; I find that the first taste slightly sour, but after that it's very refreshing plain.

> NOTE: Be sure your yogurt contains live culture; I find the brands in the health food stores (where I have to go to get the whole milk yogurt anyway) have higher quantities and better quality of live culture.

Please plan out your first week in advance, choosing what fruits you'd like to try adding. Be aware that banana has a very high glycemic index (it's totally sugar); if you must eat banana (sorry – I love them, too) only eat a half as one fruit. On a more positive note, grapefruit is a sour fruit, and, large as it is, you can eat a whole grapefruit as a fruit.

As with babies getting their first foods, we introduce foods slowly so if there is a problem it is easy to identify what food caused it. Make any changes you need to your plan, and then plan out your second week, again adding new items slowly.

I realize that planning one fruit a day for seven days is no mental challenge. But remember: learning to plan what you will eat in advance gives you a great deal of *control*, and the sense of control is very important when doing battle! Start training yourself to plan your weekly food program in advance now, so that when you move to a fully balanced program you will have experience and confidence which will greatly increase your chances of success. Start learning to listen to your body; you should now be feeling recognizably better, and attention to maintaining that feeling will help you pick up a slip before you see it on the scale.

Phase Four – *Fire At Will!*

Earlier I explained that all diets work, and that all people handle different diets differently, react to different diets differently, and get different results from different diets because their bodies are different, their tastes are different, and their lifestyles are different.

What was the most successful diet you were ever on, the one you found yourself able to stick to and that you saw success with? For the next four weeks, go on that diet. **Be sure to make any alterations necessary to keep all sugars, and processed foods out of your diet**; I'm sorry if this rules out your favorite diet. If you must eat potatoes, eat them, but choose sweet potatoes, or the small red ones, and try to eat them in small quantities, infrequently. Potatoes should never be deep fried. In fact, nothing you eat should be deep fried. Tasty as it may be, the grease/flour combination is not good for your body whether weight is an issue for you or not.

Remember: you are moving from a virtually unlimited eating pattern with a very restricted food list, to a much expanded food list, requiring you to discontinue unlimited quantities of meat and cheese, and to begin to portion control your meals. Easy greens are always unlimited.

I use all the old diet tricks everybody has heard or tried at one time. Some examples are: use a smaller plate; serve only what you are going to eat (and then don't eat it all); use small utensils; put your fork down between bites; chew each bite well and enjoy each bite as you eat it; don't drink a lot with your meal, as it dilutes the digestive juices; try to eat only one concentrated item at a meal (if you are having beef, steer clear of the bread, potatoes or rice or noodles); stop eating half way through and take a break. When we eat in restaurants, I excuse myself to the ladies room. The short break gives your appestat time to register full. (Like a car gas tank, when you get back in the car after filling the tank, the gauge does not show full, but a few moments down the road it does; your stomach registers in delayed action in much the same way.) If you are a veteran dieter as I was, you already know all these tricks and then some.

I chose to stay on phase two for almost four years because I didn't want to risk slipping back. You have the imperative information I did not at the time: the yo-yo ride back up is a result of the Yeast Beast reasserting itself as you add sugar or flour or potatoes or corn, because it was never brought under control. Once the Yeast Beast is under control, any diet will finish the job for you.

In this final phase of the diet you can switch diets as many times as you like for variety or 'staying power'; just be sure you stay on any one diet for a **minimum of four weeks**, and be **sure to Yeast-proof the diet** by making food changes to eliminate all sugars, and white complex carbohydrates (white rice, white potatoes, flour, corn).

Also at this phase it is time to start moving into *eat to live and live to eat* days. Basically, the terms are self explanatory: are you eating to nourish and fuel your body, or are you eating because it's *good*?

Eat to live days are very light for us. We graze through the day on small amounts of food to keep hunger away, and nourish the body. We don't do sit down meals on those days; though we might sit down to share leftover lamb chops, or split a tuna sandwich, we don't cook meals. We certainly don't starve ourselves. We graze on cereal, on fruit, on peanut butter 'lollipops' (peanut butter on a spoon), on cashews… it doesn't matter what we eat on those days, as we are eating small amounts of one kind of food at a time, but we do try to stick to cereal as the focal food. Most cereals are around 100 calories a cup. We eat a handful (approximately ¼ cup) and go do something else; we are getting about thirty calories at a grab. Cereal allows us to get sustenance, vitamins, and a variety of flavor readily available with no preparation, and it is fast and convenient to keep cereal in large flip lid containers so grabbing a handful is easy. If you are on maintenance it's a nearly perfect food for a grazing day.

On live to eat days, we eat whatever we want; often we use these days to let Edward loose in the kitchen (he's an outstanding chef!) or to eat out at a local restaurant. We do watch our portions, though. Often we will order appetizers only, or order one meal and split it. Most nights Edward will cook two steaks or a whole chicken, but we know that we will wind up splitting half and having a meal from the rest on the next day.

One of the tricks we utilize is to prepare single food meals; we'll have lamb chops, but either alone or with greens. Or we'll have a pasta and sauce, but no meat or cheese. Some days we graze on *only* fruit or cereal (not both) all day. One of the bonuses of concentrating on one food type for the day is the break it gives your digestive system, which does not have to fight trying to digest a mixture of foods, each of which requires different enzymes to be digested. Another benefit is that you give your body a full day shot of food choices which contain minerals and trace elements that your body needs, but does not get on a daily basis.

The next chapter deals with how foods work, and the many theories of how to make food work for dieters; many of our tricks come from pieces of these diet theories.

Chapter 15
How Foods Work

There is a labyrinth of commandments about food from different perspectives. While some are so ridiculous they are easily dismissed, such as diets with single item food lists (e.g. only eat hard boiled eggs for two weeks), diets restricting calories to starvation levels, etc., the number of sane sounding and well researched diets available is, as we say in the mold business, TNTC—Too Numerous To Count. And yet many of them not only conflict with each other, but sometimes absolutely contradict each other. How can they all work? And how do you cull the good information from each diet to grab the best of the best?

One popular concept is the food combining concept; several diets are based on these tenets. The basic rules of the diet are to eat fruit only by itself, only in the morning, and never after eating other foods, never eat protein and carbohydrates at the same meal, never mix dairy with grain or protein, and avoid mixing protein and fats. I have a friend who lost a lot of weight a combining based diet and she swears by it.

Another popular concept is to dispense with three meals a day and to eat five small ones. There's a lot of validity to this idea. The body gets weighted down by big meals; just look at all the holiday meals you've ever had where you actually had trouble getting up from the table, or had to loosen your waistband. (Or maybe, like I used to be: when you know you're going to eat a large meal you choose to wear something loose. Talk about programmed overeating!)

There are diets built around body pH. They counsel you to balance your acid and alkaline consumption. The body likes to retain an even and balanced pH. Some foods (tomatoes, acid fruits, meats, coffee, and cigarettes) are acidic in your body. Apples, greens, cereals, etc. are much more on the base end of the pH scale.

A few diets promote keeping your foods in an 80-20 relationship. They say to keep 80% of your plate filled with veggies, and 20% with protein, and then to eat only 80% and leave 20% on your plate. Once the Yeast Beast is under control, this works well for many.

Stay in the Zone: *The Zone* is a published diet promoting a balance of food groups. This diet, which is not a low carbohydrate diet, contains healthy recommendations like eating regular meals and snacks, lots of fruit and vegetables and healthier fats like olive and canola oil, and keeping these foods in specific percentages of your diet.

Have a ready-made canned shake three times a day. *Have you read the ingredients on these?* The four main ingredients are skim milk, sugar, fructose, and cocoa: in other words, milk (with milk sugar), sugar, sugar, and sugar. Other ingredients include various vegetable oils, emulsifiers, and an added vitamin blend. One canned shake contains twelve grams of protein, slightly less than what you'd obtain drinking the same amount of 1% low-fat milk. This same shake contains thirty-eight grams of carbohydrates, twenty grams more than if you drank the equivalent amount of 1% low-fat milk (the additional carbs come from the added sugar). You would be better off putting a cup of milk into a blender with some fresh fruit or instant coffee.

Replace two meals a day with a bowl of cereal and milk. This diet was first advertised by Kellogg's, for their *Special K*. The diet works as follows: eat two bowls of *Special K* cereal and a regular, sensible dinner meal and you will lose up to two to three pounds per week. This is a simple, decreased calorie diet. By following a regimen of decreased calorie consumption, any food specific diet will work. *Special K* is one of the healthier cereals out there and an excellent choice as a breakfast meal, but even Kellogg's only suggests doing this for two weeks, not for life. Focusing diet in such a narrow manner with such a decreased caloric intake is not sustainable for many people in the long-term, and not balanced or healthy enough for a permanent food program. In addition, it brings up the issue of the body's natural response to you lowering calories is to lower your metabolism, which is the very last thing you want to happen. Doing cereal all day every few days is healthy, and gives your body a break.

Eat no red meats or animal fats to avoid cholesterol problems and possible stroke or coronary. Hey, wait; so what about this diet of only protein? Possibly the most difficult diet theory to understand is how when you eat only protein and fat your cholesterol does not go up, and in fact seems to go down. I would suggest for a clear understanding of this chemistry you look into Dr. Diane Schwartzbein's book, The *Schwartzbein Principle*; she does an excellent job of making this understandable. I had a great deal of success utilizing what I learned in Dr. Schwartzbein's book, and suggest that if you just don't know where to begin, you start by purchasing her book.

The problem with most diets is that most of us just don't understand the chemistry of food and the human body. While I do not prescribe to any one tenet with religious fervor, I believe many of these tenets to be true. I think fruit should be eaten alone, and rarely eaten dried; I think protein and grains or starches should not be mixed. I think alcohol and nicotine should be declined. I think sugar should not be allowed to pass one's lips. Do I *live* by these rules? *Are you kidding?* But I do keep them in mind, and I do utilize each of them as and when it suits what I'm doing. Flexibility is an important concept in weight control.

What I do with these ideas is take them as they are: ideas. I take the sound ones. Of course I ignore them about as often as I follow them, but they are good guidelines for maintenance.

If you are going to try new foods on maintenance, knowing pitfalls like protein and starch making a hard to digest mess (how awful do you feel after Thanksgiving dinner?) can give you small areas of boost to your addition of foods. Sure, have a slice of bread; but have it with an all veggie filling, or a soup.

Many people criticize Atkins and other all (or mostly) protein and fat diets as being hard on the kidneys and raising cholesterol. I am not a doctor or a chemist, but I know that the people who research these things repeatedly report that when protein and fats are consumed *without the presence of carbohydrates*, cholesterol problems do not result, and in fact many patients (including me) report their cholesterol counts dropped while on the diet.

By the way, there are two types of cholesterol, the good kind and the bad kind. You get the good kind when you exercise. In the last few years research has been reporting that it is the good cholesterol number which is most important.

Dr. Schwartzbein's Principle, the South Beach diet, the Mediterranean diet, the Sonoma Diet, the Paleolithic Diet—these are all variations on a theme. Basically what they say is eat *a lot* of vegetables, and some fruit and some protein and little dairy. Some count it by grams, some by measurements or counts. The formulas vary but the message is the same: balance, moderation. Joseph Hall (1574–1656) said, "Moderation is the silken string running through the pearl chain of all virtues."

What does YOUR body like?

The key to the answer is *your* body. What kinds of food does *your* body want, need, do well on? Ask your mother what you liked best as a child. I have a niece who loved vegetables so much that we had to hide the baby food green beans from her until she ate the meat. I can also tell you that I have always eaten all the meat on my plate before barely touching anything else. My body likes protein. My Beast likes sugar.

What works for me for weight loss is a diet that involves lots of protein and very little sugar. I have a friend who just has to have her potatoes and pasta. She can go weeks without a piece of meat or fish, as long as she has her pasta. She doesn't have cheese with her pasta, nor bread. She can down a huge bowl of pasta and sauce for dinner several times a week and never gain a pound. I can eat this way occasionally while in maintenance, but as a weight loss campaign, it would surely backfire on me.

You can determine what works for you by going back in your dieting history and looking at the various diets you attempted, discarded, hung with, found success with; you can review how you felt on each, and where your hunger level and your cranky level were.

The cranky level is an important and often neglected issue. Feeling deprived will make you cranky. Work your diet, whatever the choice, so that you feel filled (but not full), and satisfied (not stuffed). Make what you eat appear attractive, and take time to notice eating it, tasting it, enjoying it.

If you have difficulty trying to decide what is best for you, try doing a little WWW research on food combining, protein diets, and vegetarian diets – look them all up and try each for a few weeks. Your body will surely tell you when it is not happy; you will have to look for more subtle clues to notice when it *is* happy. Do an assessment of your skin: its color, texture, elasticity, etc. Do this after a week on any diet and see if your body is showing you it likes it or not. Let the scale assist you in making your determination. While not wanting to get too personal here, do let the frequency of your bowel movements have a vote in what diet works; you will be happier with this health wise in the long run.

Again: learn to listen to your body. Don't be afraid to try new ideas. Ask others to share their experiences; in fact, you can find these on the WWW without having to ever actually talk to anyone about it. If you do a WWW search on **diet blogs**, you will get a lifetime supply of reading material about other people's experiences with dieting.

Our websites, beautyandtheyeastbeast.com and ijustblewup.com both offer links to diet.com. At diet.com they understand the varied requirements and styles of different people in different circumstances and they are set up to assist you in determining which diet will best suit your needs and preferences.

Once you have cleared your body of the Yeast Beast infestation, and you are comfortable that it's safely being kept in check, you can go on whatever form of maintenance you want, provided 1- you don't binge out on sugar and flour (which will over time give the Yeast Beast what it needs to re-infest), 2- that you continue to take your probiotics and do quarterly anti fungal cleanses, and 3- that if you have need to take antibiotics due to illness, you slam the Grapefruit Seed Extract or Candidate for thirty days; personally, when I have to take antibiotics I not only go full bore on the anti fungals and probiotics, I put myself back on the high acid, Phase One diet (Chapter 12) for however long I'm taking the antibiotics plus another week. If I have advanced notice of planned antibiotic use, as in scheduled surgery, I start the regimen a week prior to taking the antibiotics.

There is also a prescription pill called Diflucan, which is used to treat Candidiasis (also known as thrush or Yeast infection). These include vaginal infections, throat infections, and fungal infections elsewhere in the body, such as infections of the urinary tract, peritonitis (inflammation of the lining of the abdomen), and pneumonia. Diflucan is also prescribed to guard against Candidiasis in some people receiving bone marrow transplants, and is used to treat meningitis (brain or spinal cord inflammation) caused by another type of fungus. In addition, Diflucan is now being prescribed for fungal infections in kidney and liver transplant patients, and fungal infections in patients with AIDS. Diflucan is a broad spectrum anti fungal; therefore, it wipes out Fungi in the body across the board. Diflucan has a good reputation and you can certainly discuss this with your physician if you are going into a period of antibiotics. Do be aware that Fungi are very adept at mutating to make the colony immune to attack; this is why we alternate anti fungals. Remember, I am not a doctor or a health professional. Please consult your health practitioner on this issue.

I've already touted some of the benefits of cereal. When I'm on maintenance, one of my favorite tricks, as I've mentioned, is to do eat-to-live cereal *only* days. There are a number of whole grain or mostly whole grain cereals on the market now, thanks to the food industry's dedication to providing just about anything in any form that anyone could want. What I do is just graze on a handful of cereal anytime I get hungry throughout the day; I never eat enough to be full, just to quiet the hunger. I do eat cereals that contain sugar and of course flour; at maintenance I am no longer controlled by the Yeast Beast and these foods in these amounts are not a threat to Yeast Beast control; also remember I am not eating like this every day. I usually avoid the really sugary ones; you know the ones I mean. My favorite dry cereals are Cheerios (oat flour), and Spoon Size Shredded Mini Wheats (high fiber). I eat a lot of hot steel cut oatmeal, in small servings, with no added sugar or cream. (Regular Quaker oatmeal is excellent. Steel cut oatmeal is the least processed, and therefore has more vitamins and more fiber. Do not use quick or instant oatmeal as these have both been too finely processed.) General Mills is doing an outstanding job of offering a large variety of cereals utilizing whole grains, and many are 100%, whole grain. By the way, in case I was not clear: cereal grazing days are dry cereal only. We never mix cereal and milk.

I also love Raisin Bran, Cranberry Almond Crunch, and Crackling Oat Bran; however, these are considerably higher in sugar content, so I act accordingly and balance and moderate my choices. On these days we consume as much cereal we feel like, grazing in small amounts, and then have a very light dinner of protein and salad. Do make sure if you do this that you leave a few hours between your last cereal and your dinner. I am not a fanatic about food combining, but I know the stomach prefers getting the steak without cereal already there.

Please feel free to e-mail me personally if there's anything specific I can tell you; do remember I am not a physician, and do not give medical advice. My e-mail address is: Beauty@Beautyandtheyeastbeast.com.

Chapter 16
Setting up Housekeeping

You just have to hand it to the food industry; they have done an outstanding job of making available to the public every kind of food one could ask for, and in almost every way: low fat, low carb, etc. and they have been consistently responsive to changing public needs and desires in a timely fashion.

If your kitchen is anything like mine was, it's a Yeast Beast heaven. Getting rid of the cookies or chips or potatoes or bread and spaghetti and noodles is obvious; you might cringe tossing it all out, but no matter how much or little what you discard cost when you bought it, it will be well worth not having it around as you embark on this program.

If you are one of those people who keep a well stocked pantry, and what you have to dispose of is useable and unopened, you might donate it to a women's shelter or other charity as opposed to throwing it away.

You need to learn to be a serious label reader.

Start with your cabinets. If you know any item contains flour, sugar (any –ose, all artificial sweeteners, too), it gets tossed. Read the labels before you throw things out. It will give you good practice (it's a lot easier to read labels in the supermarket if you are really familiar with what information is where on the label; labels are standardized.)

What you learn about what is contained in the things that have been staples in your kitchen will probably surprise you, and hopefully give you food for thought.

When you check labels, be sure to check serving size. Though it may seem redundant, the first thing you check should be *just what is the serving size*? Often what is packaged as a single unit is shown in the fine print to be two or two and a half servings; what says 80 calories a serving may be 160 or 200 for the bottle/box/bag.

How much protein, fat, Trans fat, carbohydrate, and sugar does it contain? What is the sodium level? (Did you know high sodium foods can make you retain water, which makes it harder to lose weight, and that high sodium levels can be harmful to your heart?) What nutrients are you getting for your calories? Are you getting any fiber at all?

Read the labels on *everything*. Mustard is a great seasoning because it has virtually no calories, no carbohydrates, no sugars, and lots of taste. Do be careful not to overdo it, though, as it does contain vinegar, which the Yeast Beast likes.

Be ready for surprises. Ketchup is a *very* high sugar content item, and needs to be banned from your kitchen. (Of all the things I've ever given up, ketchup was one of the hardest for me; I think it was a double whammy combination of my allergies to sugar and vinegar and the Yeast Beast's love of both of them.) Most soups, innocent as they seem, even consommé, contain sugar and wheat. Be especially careful in ordering prepared things like soup, stews, and sauces in restaurants; you just don't know what they put in for flavor, filler, or thickening agent.

After you have cleared your cabinets, take on the refrigerator. My advice is to empty the fridge completely except for butter and mustard and go shopping. For the first two weeks, the rules are simple: eat all the protein you can, and have salad with it. Remember no salad dressings; they are sugar hideouts. Use mayo or mustard, or mix up a mayo-mustard mix. Try plain lemon juice, or lemon juice with olive oil. Again, vinegar is a Yeast Beast food, so use sparingly; Balsamic vinegar contains sugar, so, yummy as it is, it is a double whammy; I am very stingy with it.

Apple Cider Vinegar, if it is of good quality and bottled raw, is actually healthy for you. The reported cures from drinking are numerous: allergies (including pet, food and environmental), sinus infections, acne, high cholesterol, flu, chronic fatigue, acid reflux, sore throats, contact dermatitis, arthritis, and gout. Apple Cider Vinegar also breaks down fat and is widely used to lose weight. (Remember the Apple Cider Vinegar/Sea Kelp diet?) It has also been reported that a daily dose of apple cider vinegar in water has soaring blood pressure under control in two weeks! If you can get over the unusual taste of apple cider vinegar, you will find it one of the most important natural remedies in healing the body.

Cheese is an acceptable protein/fat (it's a mix of both) so don't be afraid to stock several kinds; try new cheeses! There are many varieties of regular cheese in the supermarkets, and specialty stores carry a large variety of cheese you won't see in the supermarkets. In the four years I was on protein, I ate at least a half pound of cheese every day; most days I ate more. Do be cautious, though, as cheese can be constipating.

Buy fresh meat. Be prepared to cook enough meat to provide leftovers for snacking and small meals. Remember that you want to graze on protein all day. We find that cutting up leftovers before we put them away after a meal makes them easy to grab in small amounts throughout the day. I often prepare two or three times as much meat, poultry, or fish as we intend to eat just to ensure appropriate protein availability. We eat a lot; very little goes to waste (or to waist!)

> ## *There is nothing that will put you off a diet faster than being hungry and not being able to find something that meets your needs.*

Hard boiled eggs can be a lifesaver. I used to boil up two dozen at a time. I took two or three to work with me every day, ate them peeled with a drop of salt or mustard, used them to make egg salad, or tossed them into salads; they truly are as advertised: an incredible edible.

Be wary of the deli section. Most of the selections there are not on the Phase One diet, and should probably not be eaten while you are losing. Deli meats contain a large number of additives, and high quantities of nitrates; those hot pastrami sandwiches you loved as a kid will literally kill you as a senior citizen. Stick to the one meat kind of deli: turkey, roast beef, ham, chicken, and the sliced cheeses, and avoid the salamis, bologna, and processed varieties.

I once had trouble understanding why I stopped losing after a job change. I was having my daily half pound of sliced turkey and quarter pound of cheese for lunch, something I'd been doing for almost a year. One day I asked to see the label on the turkey; it contained 2% sugar. If you are eating eight ounces of turkey for lunch, you are consuming 226 grams of turkey. Two percent of 226 grams is 4.5 grams. This means you are ingesting 4.5 grams of sugar, or a full teaspoon; that's a lot of sugar for lunch on a diet that needs to remain sugar free to combat the Yeast Beast! I switched to the roast beef and the weight began coming off again.

Don't misunderstand me; the turkey packager was not hiding a teaspoon of sugar in a portion of turkey. First of all, the FDA labeling reported that there was less than one gram (<1gm) in a serving. Remember, my serving was approximately a half pound, which was 4.5 times what they called a serving. In addition, sugar is often used as a preservative, and, as such, particularly in quantities of less than a gram per serving, is much safer for you than most other preservatives used. It is incumbent upon us as we battle the Yeast Beast to be vigilant and obtain the information we need to maintain our requirements and restrictions. I applaud establishments such as Whole Foods Markets, which place item content information on their deli price markers, making this easier for us.

Roast beef usually has no sugar added; there are also a few deli turkey roasts that do not include it. Do not be afraid to ask the person behind the counter to let you read the label. I avoid ham because it not only has sugar (a lot more than the processed turkey) but a high salt content as well, but most people on this diet easily tolerate ham as one of the unlimited proteins.

Many delis offer turkey off the frame; this is safe for you, and a good choice. Much of the sliced deli turkey in the large packages is processed; turkey off the frame may be seasoned, but it is turkey as it comes naturally. Sometimes I have them slice it, and sometimes I ask them to just cut off a two inch slice, which I can cut up and make turkey salad or stir fry meals with. They can cut any meat about an inch thick for you; simply ask them to set the blade on the widest setting and make one big slice.

Always, always, always have protein available to you with no preparation time required during the first and second phases of this program!

Canned tuna and salmon are a lifesaver. It doesn't matter if it is packed in water or oil. Sunkist now even makes tuna in foil pouches and individual sized cans with pull tabs, which both travel easily and require no can opener. If you like sardines, they are also unlimited, and the oil in them, as that in salmon, is particularly good for you. Canned tuna, sardines, and salmon (I only buy skinless/boneless sardines and salmon) can be eaten straight from the can, turned into a salad spread, crumbled into salad. Faux sandwiches/wraps can be made with large lettuce leaves; sometimes I use two slices of cheese instead of bread and put my sandwich filling between them. You are only limited by your time and imagination.

Coffee and tea: many diets tell you to avoid them. I think it's a individual, and personal, issue. There are conflicting studies about the ills and benefits of coffee, and it has been studied and debated for years. Caffeine does tend to raise your appetite a little, but for many having a cup of coffee or tea is relaxing and this is important to controlling your appetite. Recent research suggests that geriatric patients who have been lifetime coffee drinkers have less problem with dementia. As far as this program is concerned, and as long as you drink either without sugar or cream, I take no stand on the relationship between coffee/tea and health. For the purposes of Yeast Beast control and diet, they are fine in unlimited amounts. Again, I am not a physician; you might want to ask your doctor to make recommendations for you on your caffeine intake based on the medical information s/he has about you and your health needs.

Minute Maid makes frozen bottles of lemon and lime juices which are fresh squeezed, as opposed to reconstituted. I use these to slightly flavor bottled water. The diet allows two teaspoons of lemon or lime juice a day, and the little kick it gives a bottle of water has made that treat go the furthest. I also use it on salads, either alone or with olive oil. Okay, so sometimes I exceed two tablespoons a day; if that is the hardest fall anyone takes off this wagon no one will ever get hurt.

String cheese comes in individually wrapped packets; they now also have cheddar cheese packaged that way as well. The string cheese is preferable, as it is mozzarella; cheddar is an aged cheese, and some people have a problem with the mold when working on getting rid of the Yeast Beast. I personally had no problem with any cheese, and ate them, all kinds of them, in huge quantities (minimally a half pound a day) while living on straight protein/salad. It is important to note that when I moved to more varied eating, the unlimited quantities of protein and cheese were immediately discontinued. When you eat only protein the body chemically reacts differently than when you eat protein with other foods, and, in addition to the way it effects your cholesterol, it also effects you in a way that disbands the law of calories. Again, I am not a medical person, and your best source on this matter is Dr. Schwartzbein's *The Schwartzbein Principle;* she does an outstanding job of explaining this process clearly.

Do note one exception to the sugar rule: mayo has the smallest amount of sugar or honey in it. There is not enough there to cause any reaction unless you're eating mayo by the spoonful. Do not be afraid to put mayo on your protein. As I mentioned, you can try mixing mayo and mustard for a great spread or dressing. You can also mix salsa with either mayo or sour cream to make up a legal dressing or dip.

Some will tell you that any item listed more than fifth in the list of ingredients is negligible; I don't have any hard data on this, but as I know the sugar in ketchup did me in and the sugar in mayo was not perceived by my body as far as I could tell from the scale, I tend to believe there is some validity to their theory, but don't know where I would draw that line. If something has a lot of things in it, sugar could be seventh in place and still represent too much sugar; a lot of people might consider very small amounts of sugar to be negligible, and they may be right, but if you are fighting the Yeast Beast, your perspective of what "very small" means changes rapidly.

If you are going to beat the Yeast Beast you are going to have to consider the supermarket a Supply Depot. Are you stocking up to arm yourself for battle, or are you setting up a cache for the Yeast Beast?

The bill at the register may seem a little high when you first check out with your steak, chicken, ribs, cheese, lamb or whatever, but remember that you are totally avoiding the entire center of the store – all of the fresh items are along the outside ring of the store – and that you won't be putting expensive pre-processed items in your basket. It actually can come out cheaper to just buy good food!

Chapter 17
The Supplements

A healthy human gastrointestinal tract contains trillions of microbes; there are more than four hundred different species of bacteria in the human digestive tract. Most are necessary for healthy digestion and immune function.

When the micro flora balance in the colon is lost, the microbes compete for our nutrients, and their waste products overrun the intestinal tract. One of the toxins produced by Yeast is actually an enzyme which allows the Yeast to bore into the intestinal wall. The Yeast also produce other toxins which can damage the intestinal wall.

Unbalanced micro flora growth in the small intestine destroys enzymes on the intestinal cell surface, which prevents carbohydrate digestion and absorption. The last stage of carbohydrate digestion takes place at the minute projections called microvilli. Complex carbohydrates that have been broken down by the enzymes embedded in the microvilli can be absorbed properly and enter the blood stream. But when the microvilli are damaged, the last stage of digestion cannot take place. At this point only monosaccharides (simple sugars) can be absorbed because of their single molecule structure.

In the small intestine, the body should absorb the nutrients needed from what is eaten. But in the case of malabsorption, the undigested carbohydrates left in the small intestine cause the body to draw water into the intestinal tract. This pushes the undigested carbohydrates into the colon where the microbes can feast on it. This allows for even more proliferation of the unwanted microbes and continued increase in malabsorption problems.

The microbes present in the gastrointestinal tract have the potential to act in a positive, negative, or neutral manner. Microbes are not very prevalent in the stomach or upper small intestine because the environment is acidic and therefore hostile to them. However, toward the lower small intestine, where the environment is less acidic, they begin to attain higher populations, and in the colon they constitute a large portion of your colon's contents.

Probiotics are live bacteria taken to supplement the beneficial ecology of microbes in the gastrointestinal tract. They are called probiotics, the opposite of antibiotics, because they aid in creating a healthy balance of micro flora in the gastrointestinal tract.

Probiotics are an important part of the treatment for chronic Candida and other Yeast infestations. The primary use of probiotics is to restore the normal micro flora in the intestines which often occurs because of poor diet or as a result of the use of broad spectrum antibiotics, which disrupt the micro flora balance of your gastrointestinal tract.

Unfortunately, the antibiotics cannot tell the difference between pathenogenic bacteria making the body sick and friendly bacteria, which help the body to digest and function smoothly. The friendly bacteria are also what keep the pathenogenic Yeast in control. When the friendly bacteria die off, opportunistic little Beast that it is, Yeast takes the inch given and another mile as well, and increases its production of toxins in your body as it spreads.

The friendly micro-flora produces the essential byproducts of lactic acid and acetic acid, both of which help fight the growth of harmful bacteria. They also produce an acid which helps make it difficult for fungus and Yeast cells to survive and flourish in your intestines. Constipation is often corrected by ingesting large amounts of the friendly bacteria because they greatly aid in the processing of bodily wastes, decreasing the amount of time it takes for waste products to travel through your digestive system. Some people find they get constipated on the high protein phase of the diet. If you find this happening, you can increase your probiotics; you can also decrease your consumption of cheese, which is binding.

The friendly bacteria prevent harmful bacteria from taking over in the colon, where they often produce foul waste. Excess gas and chronic flatulence are often a direct result of having too few friendly micro flora in the gastrointestinal tract.

A possible side effect of antibiotics is that when they alter the bacteria in the gastrointestinal tract, decreasing the numbers of healthy bacteria, it can result in diarrhea; this is often diagnosed as Irritable Bowel Syndrome (IBS) and treated with more drugs.

Probiotics, taken during or after antibiotic therapy, can reduce or prevent the overgrowth that can result; if the antibiotics have already created an infestation condition (Yeast *is* an opportunistic Beast), they are invaluable in helping restore the balance of micro flora in your body. We utilize probiotics regularly to bolster the friendly bacteria, which assist in bringing the Yeast infestation under control. Probiotics also contain certain antimicrobial compounds which inhibit and/or destroy some of the undesirable pathogens in the intestines, including Yeast.

Generally, you should use a probiotic product which contains a mixture of live organisms and has an expiration date on the label, assuring potency. Extreme heat or freezing can kill the live cells. Food sources of probiotics include yogurt, kefir, and acidophilus milk, which all contain live cultures. Be sure to check the labeling to insure high quality live bacteria; I usually go to the local health food store for these items. If probiotics is new to you, you might want to do a little research or WWW surfing. In addition, you may want to consult your health professional before embarking on this kind of regimen.

When large doses of probiotics are first taken, mild gastrointestinal symptoms and flu-like symptoms may occur within three days. Low counts of friendly bacteria, with an increase in less desirable bacteria in the intestines can cause gas, diarrhea, constipation, mucosal irritation and contribute to the development of allergies. Another reason for these symptoms is the Yeast Beast die off. As the infestation begins to die back, the Yeast Beast in you is actually going through withdrawal: it's the Yeast Beast *Jones-ing.*

Keep in mind during the first three days that you have the Yeast Beast in apoplexy; you have the upper hand.

<u>*Be strong.*</u>

The longer you keep winning daily battles the sooner you will win the war.

It is important to utilize more than one probiotic; the Yeast Beast is clever and mutates over time, making itself impervious to single treatment solutions. We use *Threelac*, *Flora Five*, *Probio 5* and various other probiotics. It is also important to alternate anti-fungals. We use *Grapefruit Seed Extract* and *Candidate*, and find them both very effective. We take Papain (Papaya extract) to assist digestion; we also suspect it might have antifungal properties. Edward takes the papaya enzyme pills you can get at any pharmacy or health food store; I order mine on line in powder form to avoid the addition of fructose contained in the pills.

We do a Yeast Beast cleanse every three months or so, just to keep the Beast at bay. You can find links to many of these items on my website, onestopcandidashop.com, or you can do an online search for them and others. Where you get these imperative supplements is not important; it is just important that you get them and start using them as soon as possible.

Chapter 18
Laughter Really *Is* the Best Medicine

Many times being overweight leads to depression and anxiety. Coupled with a sedentary lifestyle, this is not a good emotional or physical situation for anyone. Often, the depression and anxiety lead to more eating and less movement, compounding the issue. If you are caught in this downward spiraling syndrome, try laughter.

> *"When we laugh, natural killer cells which destroy tumors*
> *and viruses increase, along with Gamma-interferon (a*
> *disease-fighting protein), T-cells (important for our immune*
> *system) and B-cells (which make disease-fighting antibodies).*
> *As well as lowering blood pressure, laughter increases oxygen*
> *in the blood, which also encourages healing."*
> *"Science of Laughter"* Discovery Health Website

Laughter has been credited with many health benefits, including stress reduction, lower blood pressure, increased energy, better breathing, and a greater ability to fight disease. It reduces harmful hormones and increases beneficial ones. Researchers estimate that laughing one hundred times is equal to ten minutes on the rowing machine or fifteen minutes on an exercise bike.

Laughing can be a total body workout: blood pressure is lowered, and there is an increase in blood flow and the oxygenation of the blood, both of which further assist healing. Laughter also gives your diaphragm, abdominal, respiratory, facial, leg and back muscles a workout as well as dozens of other muscles all over your body which flex and relax. (Good, hard laughter involves over a dozen facial muscles.) Laughter is like jogging for your insides.

New research shows that laughter can literally change your blood chemistry and help protect you from disease and depression. Researchers at Loma Linda University in Southern California report having found a physiological change at the chemical level which occurs when people laugh, and that the effects last long after the laughter subsides.

Stress constricts blood flow. Stress induces the body to produce more Cortisol, a hormone which causes us to crave food. This is why we eat when we are stressed out. So a beneficial by-product of stress-relieving laughter is that we produce less Cortisol, and therefore are less likely to crave excessive amounts of food.

Never underestimate the power of laughter.

The old slapstick comedies have stood the test of time and they make almost everyone laugh deeply and heartily. Watching your favorite comedy and laughing is good for you physically and good for your mental state. It doesn't matter if you watch The Three Stooges, classic Bob Hope or Lucille Ball comedies, reruns of sit-coms, or just funny movies; watch Road Runner cartoons for a while and just *try* not to laugh.

It doesn't make a difference whether you laugh alone or with company, but there are two possibly conflicting factors to consider about doing so: one is your comfort level in regards to letting loose your unbridled, out loud laughter in front of someone else; the other is that research shows when numbers of people watch something funny together as the whole group responds in laughter, each individual's laughter is stronger as part of the group than it is watching the same thing alone. I encourage you to try to do as much laughing *with* others as possible. My experience is that when I watch something funny I smile, or give a ha or two; rarely do I bust into sidesplitting laughter when I am alone. (You can test this for yourself: think of any comedy you saw in a theatre ever in your life that had you rolling in the isles, and rent it; watch it alone.) Any embarrassment you might feel is worth the extra laughing.

Laughing can actually turn off your

appestat temporarily; laughing for ten or

twenty seconds ten or twenty times a day

produces endorphins that satisfy

the same needs as food cravings.

Faking it works just as well. Seriously: when you make yourself laugh out loud, deeply and heartily, your body gets the exercise of a mini workout. But the side effect, partly due to the release of the endorphins, is that the laughter makes you feel as good as if you had been laughing spontaneously about something very funny. The other part is strictly mental: remember that the mind is programmable. Volumes have been written on the power of positive thinking, positive mental attitude, thought direction, self hypnosis, etc. All of them operate on the principle that the mind believes what you tell it minute to minute as you experience life.

Do remember about the unconscious 'filters' we place between us and what we see, filters configured by our experiences, upbringing, etc., as evidenced by the number of times each of us has seen something (a movie, a confrontation between two other people, a sunset…) with someone else and later, in discussion, found we had each seen the same thing very differently. How many times do police get conflicting descriptions?

In short, make time to laugh; it is good for you mentally and physically.

"Nothing is good or bad. It is thinking

that makes it so." **Shakespeare**

Chapter 19
Massage

Massage is a great way to stimulate blood flow and feel good. The act of massaging, whether by hand or with the aid of a manual or mechanical massage device, gives your arms exercise, moves your body in stretching ways, and literally shakes fat loose, disrupting its density and cohesion, allowing it to be more easily dissolved and released out of your system (particularly if you are drinking adequate water daily to flush the molecules of fat as well as toxins).

There are numerous styles of massagers available on the market and some of them can be quite elaborate and expensive, but many of them are inexpensive. The mechanical (electric) massagers work well and are especially good for the legs; they are available with a long arm that bends like an elbow and wrist, with a rotating head, which together enable you to reach all the parts of your body, and encourage your stretching.

Mechanical devices are not necessary, though; your hands can reach most of the parts of your body and they do the work just as well, plus you get the additional benefit of strengthening your hands, and keeping them limber to stave away arthritis. It would be ideal to utilize both methods in tandem.

Manual foot massagers, often wood or hard plastic, may be a Godsend for many of the obese in that they can manipulate them with their feet for the benefits of circulation and muscle awakening even if the most no-exercise exercise is found difficult because of body weight or physical condition. We recommend foot rollers for anyone: as you run your feet back and forth over the foot rollers, you move your legs (your legs do not get any real exercise, but the muscles are used and stimulated and this prepares them for work and helps raise your metabolism), relax your feet, stimulate nerve endings, increase circulation, which helps move good things and bad things where they need to be, and massage the organ and system components of your body, as explained below. If you have a supportive partner, offer to trade massages with him/her.

You can purchase hand and foot reflexology charts at most health food stores and on line. They even make little gloves and socks that have the charts imprinted for 'spotting' each area. Each part of the palms on our hands and the soles on our feet correspond to the myriad of organs and systems in the body. While this is not an exact science, it is a time honored and proven means of stimulating all the organs and nerves in your body.

Don't be concerned at first with which part of your body you are working on: an all over massage will hit everything. If you never investigate the charts at all and just do foot and palm massage you will reap benefits without involving charts and locations. But if this does interest you, as you become familiar with the charts, you can pick areas you'd specifically like to target and work on them.

This is an exercise you will find easy to do which can be done almost anywhere, almost anytime. Paying attention to the palms of your hands and the soles of your feet, rub in gentle circles in each area of the palm/sole for a few moments. Run your massaging hand down the ridges on the back surface of your hands along the metacarpals (the five cylindrical bones extending from the wrist to the fingers) and down the ridges on the tops of your feet along the metatarsals (the five cylindrical bones extending from the heel to the toes); there are important energy grids here which are assisted by stimulation. Again, this is not my area of expertise, but I can tell you that getting the energy of your body unblocked is important to physical and mental health. You might want to do your own research in this area, or speak to someone who is into holistic health.

There is nothing that soothes the body and the soul like a good massage.

You can start your massage on any area of the body: arms, legs, thighs, neck/shoulders, abdomen, or derrière; there is no right place to begin. Work each area for a few minutes, rubbing, squeezing, and kneading your self in areas where there are visibly fat deposits. If you're where I was when I started, *everywhere* was an area of visible fat deposits. Move from one area to the next, making sure if you work on an area on one side of your body, you do the same area on the other side before choosing a new location.

If you like to bathe, as opposed to showering, you can do self massage in the tub; it is very relaxing. It was torturous for me to take baths after I reached a certain size because I could not lie there for that long without having to acknowledge what my body looked like; heck, even if I tried to keep the surface covered in bubble layer, my body displaced so much water that, without overfilling the tub, my whole body would not submerge at one time. It was personally embarrassing, even though no one else ever knew, and it was a sad loss, because I had always loved a long, relaxing bath, and had never taken one since then, until I started working on Phasing and the mirror. Now I use the tub as a forced time to just be with my body.

Stimulating massage is healthful. A vigorous massage will burn a few calories, get your blood flowing, help flush toxins, help you to feel good, and will get you started on a more healthful lifestyle.

The power of the mind is an amazing thing. I have already mentioned my belief in the possibilities available to us through positive thinking, positive mental attitude, thought direction, self hypnosis: I am surely no authority in this area, and am not saying here that I believe you can think yourself thin, but I do believe that putting your mind's concentration on the removal of fat deposits on your body in a focused manner has got to help.

Your mind talks to and with you all day. It chastises you when you cheat. It has something to say about most people, even if you never verbalize these things. Your mind fills your head with thoughts all day in rapid fire without much cohesiveness to the topic of the thought. Choose things you want your mind to believe or do, and direct the topic of thought in your head whenever possible. Keep telling it until it hears; eventually your mind will grasp the thought and decide that the whole thing was its idea and then you're home free.

> ### *"For Satan finds some mischief still*
> ### *For idle hands to do."*
> ### *Isaac Watts (1674–1748)*

Tell yourself you love to move. Tell yourself you know when you're hungry and when it's really water that you need. Tell yourself you prefer (*anything good for you*) to (*anything not so good for you*).

When you hear your mind disparaging your fat it is time to program it with new thoughts on the matter. Acknowledge what weight you've lost, what muscle you've gained. Give it a mental picture of what you will look like twenty pounds less, and tell it you are showing it a current picture; these are just in-your-head exercises in giving direction. Remember that left to its own devices, the mind will tell you things that may not be in your best interest. It certainly will speak to you in ways that reinforce any negative images and feelings you have about yourself, and those which are the remnants of someone else's opinion dumped on you, whether on occasion or historically; we all have specific moments and those over time (or ongoing) which leave remnants and the remnants quietly rub in the back of our minds, like sand in an oyster, until they become coated with a hard surface. Unfortunately, we are not making pearls, but self degradation stones.

Massage yourself.
It feels good; it works

Rest and relaxation: these are important tools to the success of any health program, and they are commonly considered important for mental health. Do get enough rest, and invest some time in relaxation techniques and breathing techniques for relaxation.

There are two simple techniques I will pass along to you here. Neither is original; both are time honored techniques. Please consider doing some research on your own for other techniques, methods, and programs for breathing and relaxation. A plethora of information is available on the WWW, as well as at your public library. Even the local high school should have enough information on this subject to allow for a good start.

Relaxation: Lie comfortably on your back. Close your eyes. Starting at your toes, mentally tell yourself (you know, talk to yourself in your head) that your toes are relaxing. Feel them relaxing. Work your way up the body, doing one small section at a time (toes, arch, heel, ball of foot, ankle, lower calf, upper calf, etc.) and telling yourself that area is relaxing. Do one leg then the other. Next, relax your arms, again, one small portion at a time (fingers, palm, wrist, etc.) Then relax your torso, then your neck, and then your head. Don't be surprised if you fall asleep the first few times; in fact, I often use this technique when I'm having trouble getting to sleep, and often don't make it further than my legs. The important thing is the time spent actively working on putting your attention on your body and relaxing it.

Breathing: Sit comfortably in a chair with your back well supported and your feet flat on the ground. With your left hand, use your index finger to hold closed your left nostril. With your eyes closed, breathe in slowly to the count of four through the right nostril. Hold this breath for the count of four. Switch hands, closing the right nostril and releasing the left. Next, slowly release the breath through the left nostril to the count of four. Without moving your hands, breathe in through your left nostril, slowly to the count of four. Switch hands and place your left index finger on the left nostril and release the breath through the right nostril. Repeat the process. Do this for as long as you can whenever you feel the need to collect yourself or relax. By the way, next time you are heading out to face a difficult meeting or phone call, just a few repetitions of this exercise beforehand will help you remain much more in emotional control and to think more clearly through the conversation. I can tell you there has been many a time I took a moment in the stall before leaving the ladies room to center myself in this manner.

We tend to take our bodies so much for granted. We run them on empty; we run them on Twinkies; we run them without sleep, or exercise. When we are fourteen years old, we can pull an all-nighter and function the next day. When we are fifty-something, we just don't get to do that any more without paying dearly. One of the most important things we can do as we turn our lives around is to start showing ourselves that we are important and valuable to ourselves, and that we are going to take care of ourselves.

Chapter 20
The Time Factor

All of life's little chores take time; generally, most take more time than you want or expect. Major undertakings are just humongous chores. Getting healthy, staying healthy, and recovering from obesity all take time. You need to take an honest look at yourself and see how far out of shape you have become over the past however many years or decades; what is your weight and fitness level now compared to when you were in high school? What was it when were you at your best, and how do you compare now?

If you have never been in shape, the way I had never been in shape, you will need to find an alternate model to focus on besides yourself to determine how fit you would like to be, and at what weight. Don't look to superstars. Look at people you know, or look through a high quality magazine which features non-model, non-celebrity, real people. There are several good ones out there.

You have two choices: a healthful old age or advanced infirmation (see Chapter 2) and physical misery. No matter how much time it is going to take you, you can spend the time on yourself now promoting good health, or spend the time later tending to your poor health.

The time factors you face are those of controlling the Yeast Beast, losing the weight, eating properly for you, and getting strong.

We evolved as an active species, designed to run and climb. In the scheme of evolution, it's just not all that long ago that if you couldn't run you wouldn't survive; this is the way we are built, and how we evolved.

Our bodies were designed to carry a workload. There was certainly Yeast historically before the Industrial Age, but I couldn't find anything about Yeast infestation back anywhere nearly that long ago. Work moves blood. Work removes fat from muscle tissue. Work makes us sweat, and sweat removes toxins. Work keeps our digestive track moving. You just don't get Yeast infestations when you are working hard enough every day, six days a week, for ten hours a day to move that much blood, remove that much fat, remove that many toxins, and keep everything moving along at a clip that removes the opportunity for Yeast to get out of control.

I imagine that if anyone were willing to dig ditches eight hours a day s/he would lose weight irrespective to how much of what food s/he ate in what combination, at what time of day. I imagine that if anyone were willing to spend eight hours a day working (remember, working makes us sweat) on Godzilla, our *Versa Climber*, s/he would lose weight irrespective to food consumption as well.

I surely don't suggest anyone dig ditches or pump on Godzilla for eight hours a day!

What I am getting to is that our bodies have to work; it's part of the mechanics of our bodies. Animals which were bred to work do not remain healthy for long if they do no work and eat more than they need to eat for their activity level to be healthy. Most of us as overweight and obese or morbidly obese people do little to no exercise. (Many of us have had periods of avoiding activity as much as possible.)

If we are to be healthy, we need to work enough and eat right enough to balance our micro flora and keep strong for our weight. The more you are willing to work hard and eat right, including supplements, the faster you will be in shape and the better shape you will be in. It's a sliding scale. On one end there is 100% work (eight hours of sweat) and 100% correct eating, and on the other end of the scale is 0% work and 0% correct eating. Each of us has an idea of what we want for ourselves in terms of levels of work and intake. No one *wants* to be at 100% ,100%. But no one wants to be at 0%, 0% either. Each of us has an imaginary balance point in mind. We also have the reality point of where we are currently. What is in our hands is the choice to make the move from where we are to where we want to be.

In the early 1950's much of America was rural. Large groups of working children labored on family farms all across this nation. After the urbanization of America, American children went from physical chores on the ranch or farm to go make your bed and then you can go watch television, and then to video games, portable video games, music devices, and the WWW. If you grew up on television and video games and have never been strong, you are going to need a serious program and length of time to recover from obesity and build strength.

The Yeast Beast will not like it when you start to move. He likes your metabolism nice and slow.

The time factor on the Yeast Beast war is a function of the level of activity you choose, how well you stick to the food program and the utilization level of the supplements. I lost 125 pounds in just under a year, with no exercise program; I lost the entire 180 pounds (I added exercise after the first 125 pounds) in a total of fourteen months. If you have this much to lose, this is a lofty goal to shoot for, but certainly I am proof that it is do-able. Do remember that for two years I ate nothing but protein and salad and I was religiously fanatical about it. I wouldn't even take vitamins unless I was sure they were sugar and wheat/gluten free. In the second two years, I cheated and enjoyed it thoroughly, but I cheated infrequently, and went right back to the program afterwards.

If I knew then what I know now...

Had I had this guide when I started, I would have found a way to make movement and exercise part of my program from the beginning. I have no doubt that even if exercise didn't improve my rate of weight loss (though I absolutely believe it would have done so), it surely would have improved my level of fitness and strength; yo-yo dieting takes a lot of muscle and burns it as we starve ourselves (calorically and/or nutritionally) on various diets. When we gain the weight back, we don't gain it back as muscle, but as fat. I work out twice a day these days: once for the day, and once to make up for one of the only-God-knows-how-many days of no exercise for the best part of fifty years.

You may find that your body responds really well to a new routine and that this change of lifestyle becomes enjoyable. Once the Yeast Beast starts coming under control and the weight starts to come off, your energy level will go up and you will be able to get things done more quickly and easily; you are also likely to find your concentration noticeably improved.

Exercise definitely assists in minimizing the effects of a cheat. We say exercise can *legalize* cheating; this is of course just an expression, but it holds fairly true if you keep the cheats reasonable. One piece of cheesecake (my favorite cheat) isn't going to kill me or wreck my fitness unless I'm eating it daily or eating the whole cake in a short period of time.

As an aside, I only cheat with what I know to be or strongly expect to be the thick, solid, creamy, almost all cream cheese kind I like or I won't eat it, even if it was my planned cheat. I do this intentionally for me for two reasons. The first reason is that I felt from the beginning that if I am going to cheat, and if I am only get to do so infrequently, the cheat had better be worth the cost. The second reason, which is two pronged, came along as part of my psychological phasing. The first prong is actually an extension of the first reason: if I am going to eat *anything*, it is going to be worth the cost. The second prong was a lot newer for me: I am worth having the best that is within my means. That last one is still being ingrained; there is a lot of contradictory historical thought on the subject in my mind.

Back on track here. The time factor on the supplements is two fold. 1- You take the Grapefruit Seed Extract, Candidate, or other antifungal (we recommend alternating your anti-fungals every thirty days) for ninety to one hundred and twenty days. 2- You take the probiotics daily, forever; once the Yeast Beast is at bay, you can cut down taking the probiotics to two or three times a week and that will be sufficient.

YOU are in control.

The wonderful thing about this program is that you can use it to lose large amounts of excess weight and you can control just how much you lose and how fast you lose it by determining the level at which you follow the program: diet, supplements, exercise/no-exercise.

Let me be really frank here. What you put into things determines what you get out of them, generally, and this Yeast control treatment program is no different, nor is the exercise component of it. You can choose what level of fitness you want your body to be at when you have completed the Yeast treatment program and lost the desired amount of weight. If you want to be thin and soft, you can do that. If you want to be overweight but not obese, and soft *or* fit, you can do that. If you want to be thin *and* fit you can do that, to whatever level of fitness you desire.

Having said that, I need to add the following (also frank) item, particularly for the ladies, but for you guys, too. It's not an easy item, so I am just going to put it out there in a straightforward matter of fact manner. If you are in an intimate physical relationship, regardless of legal or residential status, you need to acknowledge that it is also in your hands what body you bring to the bed at night.

If you want to be beautiful or handsome and fit, you can, and it's worth it.

I know that this is a private matter, and you need to know I am in no way making any judgment calls here; this is simply several factual statements and an opinion. I debated whether or not to include it in this book for some time. The decision to include was made based on what I know about how the Yeast Beast stole the entire concept of beauty from me, my whole life long. Beauty is a woman's birthright. I don't mean that every woman is born beautiful, or that every woman *is* beautiful. But every woman has the right to look the best she can and *feel* beautiful. If the Yeast Beast has stolen that from you, too, take it back.

The level of exercise you choose (or the level of exercise at which you are able to start along with the rate that you are able to progress at) will have a distinct impact on the result when you complete your weight loss.

Chapter 21
The Economic Cost to the Victim

The economic cost of unwilling obesity to the life of the victim defies calculation. Starting with self imposed limitations and compounded by the limitations imposed by mostly covert prejudice, the effect is staggering. I had well paid positions as a public school administrator. However, I could have done much better.

The first limitations come from our ability to be willing to admit being overweight but our inability to consciously see to what extent. For those of us who are/were obese, and those of us who are/were morbidly obese, it is an additional, almost insurmountable, difficulty to acknowledge being obese, even when it turns into morbid obesity (defined by the medical profession as being more than one hundred pounds overweight), or to even let this information pass through our mental filter system into our consciousness.

*If you are reading this because someone you love has the Yeast and weight problem, do, please do for their sake, try to understand—and I know it is seemingly not understandable: It is not that they deny or pretend anything. They **<u>can not see</u>** their own reflection and give*

***an accurate description of what is being
reflected to them in terms of their size, because
their mind has stopped allowing that image in
for self protection.***

Everybody has some area of insecurity that they hide from others, cover up or minimize. I always wore bangs because I hated the way my forehead looked (it's just a little high but seemed mutant to me). My mind assumed the world not only noticed my forehead, but that it really cared and it really hated it. Covering it took away the issue.

Covering my forehead with bangs also served to minimize the input of reflection from the mirror, which diminished my ability to see that which I was critical and judgmental about when I looked at myself, which made living with my mutation easier. (This is just what happens; it is not a conscious decision or even something one is aware of.)

The brain sees and records everything. If we were conscious of everything we saw, we'd have no room left to think. The brain, on an unconscious level, most often under your conscious or unconscious direction, decides what we need to see. For example, you can live in a town for five years and never notice a real estate sign. But if you decide to buy or sell your house, you will not go anywhere until the transaction is complete and you have moved where you do not see real estate signs *everywhere you look*; it is as if you told your brain to look for them. Actually, you did. This is the way our brain works.

When we limit the input of information we allow into our mind, consciously or unconsciously, we do not get a full picture of reality. The input we allow *becomes* our reality. It is unfortunately a huge, unconscious, self-deception inside whose walls we build our lives.

When we are very overweight we cannot hide this source of insecurity and perceived judgment and criticism from others. More importantly, when we are very overweight we cannot hide this source of insecurity and our *own* judgment and criticism from *ourselves*. So the mind protects us from this pain and the unsolvable, unacceptable condition by making it invisible to us. It *limits the input* allowed. This limited input becomes our reality. We live within the walls of this literal delusion. *We do not know this.*

This unconscious self-deception, over time, forced me to work where I could pass the covert physical appearance minimum requirements. I landed a lot of jobs where casual dress was acceptable after the interview and no one really cared what you looked like as long as you were clean and presentable, met their needs and got all your paperwork in on time and with accuracy.

This self imposed, self limiting avoidance behavior cost me a much better career and thousands of dollars a year. The prejudice I encountered lead me to believe that I was the Queen of Coming In Second. This prejudice reinforced my self imposed limitations and my career went to smaller districts where the pay was much less. I was earning $75,000. a year, but I know that for the same work in a higher profile district I would have earned much more. There would also have been many other opportunities available to me, opportunities which do not exist in smaller districts.

My professional accomplishments could not be capitalized on. Public appearance required of administrators was so hard for me. There were many times I did not apply for jobs I could have done well because I knew my ability to *look right* alone disqualified me walking in the door, before the interview even happened. I can write. I have a Master's Degree in Educational Administration, a Bachelor's Degree in English, a minor in psychology, and nine educational credentials. I never pursued writing as a vocation because of the public appearance factor; my best appearance would never be good enough.

How much money do you make? Would

you be making more if you were slim, fit and

strong? Would other opportunities be available

which are out of the question now? These are

just a part of your victim costs.

The University of Michigan analyzed data on more than 7,000 men and women in their fifties and sixties in 1992, and reported that the individual net worth of a moderately to severely obese woman between the ages of fifty-one and sixty-one was about forty percent less than that of her non-obese counterpart, after statistically controlling for a number of demographic and health factors.

In 1998, a moderately to severely obese woman between the ages of 57 and 67 had an individual net worth of about sixty percent less than her non-obese peer; again, the study controlled for important demographic and health factors.

It is interesting to note that the effects of obesity for men were generally not statistically significant.

Obesity is a disease, now recognized by the US government as such. According to the Surgeon General, the nation's economic cost of obesity in 2000 was $117 billion and 300,000 deaths per year were associated with it. A 1999 report showed 61 percent of adults in the U.S. were overweight or obese. Current figures on the percentage of obese adult Americans are now being reported at about 80%. The American Obesity Association reports the number of overweight and obese Americans has increased steadily since 1960, a trend that is not slowing down.

As the prevalence of obesity has increased in the United States, so have related health care costs, both direct (preventive, diagnostic, and treatment services) and indirect (wages lost by people unable to work because of illness or disability and future earnings lost as a result of premature death). The current crisis in the insurance industry, the accompanying skyrocketing costs of services, and the resulting number of people without insurance in this country have been tremendously impacted by the medical cost of obesity, and this cost directly effects what we have to pay when we have medical needs, whether we are obese or not.

There are numerous emotional costs to the victim. Every relationship, be it family, friends, lovers, co-workers, superiors, subordinates, store clerks or the garbage man, is affected by our obesity and by the psychologically manifested symptoms. The level to which the relationship is affected varies, and the emotional pain resulting from any acknowledged affects also varies. I handled it by getting emotionally tough on the inside: I couldn't be touched emotionally. But at the same time, I was an emotional basket case if you cracked through the wall.

The emotional cost for me in terms of family came dearly. Years of being the one to "go off" over something no one else could see as having any reason to care, years of behaviors which were contentious, critical, ornery, and argumentative just cumulatively took its toll on my family relationships. My mother has told me I have always been a disappointment to her. My daughter also believes I have always been a disappointment to her, and has expressed this in many ways. No one in my family ever understood me, and, as I never understood myself nor did I ever realize that they couldn't understand me, I just spent my life not fitting in, not belonging, and pretty much just unconsciously creating chaos for unconsciously needed attention.

When I underwent the psychological aspect of Phasing, a tremendous anger was released. A veil which had been up for many, many years came down, and I saw a lot of things quite clearly. Edward was astute in grasping this period of epiphany and helping me to verbalize and work through much of it. I tried to explain to my family that something was different, but they had such a strong, well entrenched mind set of who and what I was, they were unable to see it, or even to hear it and consider it; they were not even able to see the physical differences in me beyond my initial large weight loss.

I hope you do not encounter this kind of reaction, and that you find your family supportive. Do prepare yourself, however, for the realization that the person your family has known all their lives will be different, and different families will have different tolerance levels and different levels of the ability to restructure their mind set. If you are reading this book because there is someone you care about and wish to understand and help, know that letting that person know you understand this may help them to be able to see it for the first time.

While certainly not in the serious vein of the previous paragraphs, there is one more cost (both financial and emotional) to the victim I should mention: clothing.

When you are very overweight or obese, your clothes are going to cost more. Your choices are going to be decreased. The majority of clothing I owned was chosen for the most basic of needs: it fit.

You will at some time face embarrassment in a store over clothes. Probably the least embarrassing incident, though one which happened repeatedly, was the one where the saleslady loudly announced I needed the Plus Size Department, upstairs (you know, way back in the corner), or that they don't make that item in a size that big, or to suggest that I try looking at Lane Bryant's?

You will most assuredly feel guilty or inadequate as you bypass all the sections of regular sizes on your way to the 'fat section'. (Call it Plus Size, call it Full Figure: they're all just PC (politically correct) ways of saying fat.) You may realize as I did one day, that you hadn't been in a department store for a long time; all of your clothing has been ordered on line or through catalogs.

You will settle for something for an important occasion that is not just what you had in mind. The dress I wore to my own Sweet 16 was the *only* one we were able to find that fit me and did not look matronly, as I was wearing a size 18/20.

You will choose clothes that seem to diminish the area(s) of your body you most want to diminish, and this will be more important than style or color. I once bought a dress that had an ugly print just because the color and price were okay and the way it hung hid my stomach. (That's what I thought then; right now, I'd venture to guess it didn't hide anything.).

Emotional slaps in the face, whether from an external source or an internal reaction, hurt. They are a cost as real as any financial cost, and for some, surely for me, they comprise the brunt of the cost to the victim.

Don't let the costs of the Yeast Beast hurt you. Get control of the Yeast Beast now. Take back your life.

Chapter 22
Self-Subjection: Lower Than Second Class

Failure is difficult to live with. Recurring failure is far more devastating and can lead to a morass of psychological issues, depression, and low self esteem.

For many a life of solitude is the destined future. House bound and living via the WWW is a currently existing private hell for many. Several years of this house bound lifestyle is unhealthy for anyone, but especially for the obese. There are actually cases of grossly/morbidly obese people who either live on Social Security or work from home who have eaten themselves into a form too large to get out their own door. There are actual cases of people having strokes or heart attacks and the paramedics cannot get them moved because of their weight. These are very sad and scary facts to me. I personally had an experience last year when a neighbor's husband collapsed; he landed mostly on his side. I gave him CPR while waiting for the paramedics, but it was difficult as his head was one side down and he was so obese I could not roll him from his side over onto his back.

Obesity has been in the news a great deal lately, and particularly obesity in regards to school aged children. President Clinton has recently taken on this issue. The stigma of being overweight is beginning to get worse and as it does it isolates the victim of obesity. As long as we are carrying too much weight our self-image suffers, our careers languish, and our lives become confusing.

Recurring weight loss failure after partial diet success, or *Diet Failure Syndrome,* when it is not understandable due to a lack of information, does not promote mental health;

feelings of guilt and lack of self worth blossom. We expect to be able to control ourselves, and we know others expect us to be able to control ourselves, but we can't seem to control ourselves, or even if we do it doesn't seem to help; living like this will make you extremely insecure, self-depreciating, and self-degregating.

If I can't love and respect myself, why should anyone else?

In the days of Women's Liberation, women were depicted as being subjugated, second class citizens. For better or worse, changes came about that gave women a considerably more equitable position in life. I have to tell you: if you are obese and would rather not be obese, the feelings you will have towards yourself will lead you to make yourself more of a second class citizen than any man, boss, or situation ever could.

I believe my missing makeup gene was in reality just a lack of experience brought about by years of not feeling worth trying to make myself up; I already knew, had already been programmed: I was not the beauty. I don't know how many other inadequate feelings manifested themselves in my life, but I know that there were always feelings of inadequacy, despite accomplishment, and that how I walked, how I dressed, how I talked, and how I responded in every situation was effected by it.

How long will you let the Yeast Beast control *your* life, *your* weight, *your* attitude, *your* career, *your* marriage, etc.? Take back your life. Declare war on the Yeast Beast today.

Chapter 23
It Doesn't Matter, Really

When my niece was about thirteen years old, I asked her to run down to the corner store (a convenience store) for me. She was aghast. *"I can't go there; I have no makeup on."* So? *"Well, I might meet someone I know.... I might meet someone I don't know!"* It was a very funny moment, and the phrase has been quoted in our family many times.

There is really a huge issue in this tiny story. My response of, *So?* said it all. She was thirteen, and I was thirty. At thirty I could not understand why this child would care whether or not she had makeup on for a five minute run down to the corner convenience store. At thirty, I barely cared if I had makeup on at all.

I'd throw some eye shadow and mascara on and call it makeup, and there were many days when I didn't even do that. I just didn't think it made any difference, so why bother?

While I'd been married, I really had never been in a relationship with anyone who cared if I had makeup on or not. It was something I did for special occasions. Later, it would be something I did for interviews and the beginnings of school years and for functions; it was never something I did on a regular, daily basis, never anything I did for me, and never something of any importance to me. And in hindsight, I'm willing to bet there were many more people I worked with who might disagree than agree with my assessment that no one cared what I looked like.

Don't get me wrong; I didn't run around in dirty or torn clothing. I was just a department store clearance sale/mail order catalog kind of gal (you know, if you order things by catalog, you don't have to walk around the fat store), and it is really embarrassing to admit that, and to admit that it really came down to I didn't think enough of myself to bother trying to do the best I could with what I had.

I remember vividly the moment I had my first stark realization of how I used to be in terms of clothing and makeup. Edward and I had been partners for more than six months, but we had only been involved personally for a few weeks. Makeup was something I did for Edward all the time; it had not yet become something I ever did for me.

We were having lunch out, and, before we left, I excused myself to go to the ladies room. After washing my hands, I took out my comb and fixed my hair and then put on a little lipstick; I straightened my blouse.

As I was doing so, I saw a large lady go to the sink, wash her hands, glance at the mirror and touch her hair; then she shot me a dirty look and left.

I had one of those flashing lights moments, an epiphany, an *Oh My God*, a déjà vu all over again: that was me. That was me for forty years.

Even as a teen I had distain for the girls who spent all of all passing periods in front of the mirror in the bathroom. How messed up could your hair or makeup get in fifty-five minutes in a classroom? Whatever drive they had to make themselves look good, I thought I had an area or retardation or was gene deficient. My mother will tell you I wore too much eye makeup in high school; this is true. I wore heavy black liner and mascara. But I really never wore anything else, and never wore lipstick; I'd try every once in a while to buy and use one, but the lipstick never stayed on more than a few minutes anyway, as it annoyed me into licking it off, and I wasn't going to start getting into any 'ritual' that required continuous attention.

When you look at the mirror and you feel hopeless you tend not to bother to try.

Somewhere along the way, I developed the ability to look in the mirror and *not see*. I could get dressed in the morning without even using a mirror; I'd check in the mirror before leaving that my clothes were straight, but *never mentally register* what I looked like; I'd do my hair and makeup, and never *see* what I looked like. As you know from the last chapter, this is a psychological defense mechanism of the mind.

When I look at pictures of me now from the years I was obese, and there are precious few of them, I cannot believe I actually looked like that, and that, while I knew I was overweight – a lot overweight – I never felt obese, never thought I was obese, and certainly never thought anyone else thought I was obese. (Look at the pictures on the back cover; I was obese.)

When I look at those pictures now, I am shocked. First, you must realize that there are precious few pictures of me; they were either not taken because I made myself unavailable, or they never survived my seeing them. So if a picture of me found its way to the photo album, I must have felt it was good, or at least not so bad I had to tear it or burn it (having done both in the past).

When I look at those surviving pictures now, I do not comprehend how I could *not* have been aware of what I looked like. When I look at those pictures I can remember the time and event and even the clothing I wore in them, but I am telling you God's honest truth, I never remember being that big. I walk into a restaurant now, and actually wonder how I could have not been embarrassed to do so before. I sit on restaurant chairs (the dumb café kind that are so tiny), and though I can now remember how little of me rested on them, and am aghast that at the time I never even realized it. I think back and shiver at what I must have looked like coming to my husband at night with romance on my mind (though, as I said, he was always complimentary.).

I'm not sure that the tacit approval of my weight by everyone around me did me any favor. While having had someone sit me down and make me let them mirror back to me what the world saw would have been excruciating, it would have been kinder than letting me continue in my disillusionment.

Parents, siblings, spouses, lovers, friends or fat people: if you are not trying to help them see themselves, you are letting them down. I'm not talking about telling someone they need to go on a diet. What they need is someone who will go to the mirror with them and help them to assess themselves, and then help to them move that assessment a little closer to reality. I'm talking about helping them see ways in which their behavior may be difficult. Be prepared: this may be as well received as an Alcoholics Anonymous intervention, but, just as in AA, sometimes an intervention is needed. The good news is, when the problem has been handled, the person usually is grateful to the brave soul who did it.

If you are more than fifty pounds overweight, no matter how well you carry it, you need to go look in the mirror and find out if you, too, have learned not to see. You need to understand, and I know this hurts, that everyone around you who is not fifty pounds overweight most likely sees you as fat, maybe as lazy, and certainly as having a lack of willpower and self control.

They don't understand that it's the Yeast Beast. It's not your fault; It's the Yeast Beast.

When I put on makeup now, I still do it for Edward; but now I do it for me, too. And I'm starting to learn to play with it, experiment, and try new things. I remember as a young adult thinking that if they could take female impersonators and make them gorgeous with makeup, I should be able to do something. Helena Rubinstein said there were no ugly women, only lazy ones.

Clothing is another area where years of being plus size (most of my adult life was spent in size 20-26's) left me disinterested and discouraged. My wardrobe consisted of what I could find that fit in an acceptable color/style/pattern and price. If I found a good t-shirt, or skirt or stretch-waist pants, I bought one of each color (except white or yellow or pink or any of the other light colors because light colors make you look bigger, right?). Shoes in extra wide are hard to find, and heels hurt even if you could find them in your size. I wore only flats and mostly well broken in, comfy shoes. Whenever possible, I wore jeans, a t-shirt, and tennies. I mostly didn't try. I just didn't even try.

Now I buy fewer clothes, but what I buy looks good, and is made well and fits well. I visit the cosmetic counter about once a month just to see get a tip or try a new color. I just don't leave home without makeup; *I might meet someone I know; I might meet someone I don't know!*

It's really a second adulthood.

Chapter 24
Weights

I keep talking about exercise/no-exercise. No-exercise means you don't have to do any exercise, just as it sounds. However, you *do* need to start awakening soft and unused muscles in preparation for getting fit; it is my hope that you will move from no exercise to no-exercise with wrist/ankle weights, to walking with weights, to any other form of exercise: yoga, Pilates, Tae-Bo, ballet, dance salsa, aerobics, gyms or machines; it doesn't matter what your choice of movement is, only that you move.

Ankle and wrist weights can be a life saver if you have been sedentary for a long time or just need to start moving. It can be a challenge to get into a healthy lifestyle and ankle and wrist weights are a great way to painlessly start asking your muscles to wake up.

If you haven't done any physical work beyond housecleaning in a long time, your muscles are going to need a reintroduction to work wake up call.

Wrist weights do not require that you grip the weight; the weight simply wraps around your wrist; most are held in place by Velcro straps. It is not necessary to use a lot of poundage to start. As little as a one pound weight (you would buy a two pound pair) on each wrist is enough to start on your program of weight loss and health. You can wear small weights throughout the day even at work or shopping as well as around the house and the weight will soon become so normal you won't even realize that you have the weights on. In fact, sometimes when I've been walking most of the day with my ten pound weights on under my jeans (a twenty pound pair), I take them off and it feels like my legs are floating up as I walk for a few moments before my body readjusts itself. It makes me seriously realize how easily we get used to carrying extra weight.

Many people with a weight problem also have leg and foot problems. Walking may not be available as a form of exercise. If this is the case with you, please refer to the chapter on massage. Foot massagers, both manual and mechanical, will help. If you cannot walk, massagers will help to get your blood circulating and you can leave your wrist weights on while using your foot massager. Also know that your arms are as good a source of cardiovascular and metabolic stimulation as your legs.

Using wrist weights and increasing the weight over a period of time can be evolved into a serious workout. Upper body workouts are muscle building and are easily aerobic. Movements that make your arms go higher than your heart are particularly beneficial to cardiac health.

Be careful when you are using wrist weights move slowly; refer to the instructional photos in this chapter. Do not toss or throw your arms with your weights on as you could sprain or pull a muscle or tendon. Move your weighted arms and legs slowly and with rhythm and purpose. Once you start using your wrist weights you will find that watching a movie while wearing the wrist and/or ankle weights and keeping them in motion while you enjoy the show is not difficult. Simple movements like a "wave" at a baseball game, or hula hand movements, or just making figure eights in the air will slowly tone muscle and will begin to elevate your metabolism, which is of great importance to losing weight.

Walking with wrist and ankle weights is possibly the best exercise there is. Start out with light poundage and walk for endurance. Longer walks at a moderate pace are best to start. Keep the weight on your wrist and ankles fairly equal as the balance will make walking easier; it is best to carry more weight on your wrists than on your legs, even though carrying the weight on your ankles is easier because the leg muscles are so much larger and usually in better shape than our arms. Music helps.

Any comfortable outfit will work; you do not need a wardrobe to work with weights. Don't think you need to run out and buy special workout clothing. Most often I work out on Godzilla in Danskin tights (which I wear almost all the time) with an inexpensive cotton or terry miniskirt (or just a pair of sweats) and a t-shirt or a leotard, and usually do my walking in jeans or shorts and a t-shirt.

Walking for exercise without wearing/carrying weights is of little benefit.

Stretching, kicking, doing Tai Chi, etc. while wearing ankle and wrist weights makes for great workouts which can be done at home. Furthermore, saving the cost of membership and the travel time to utilize a gym makes using inexpensive and portable wrist and ankle weights very sensible.

The cost of ankle and wrist weights is low; however, as you will be starting out with lighter weights and adding poundage, you can end up with several sets of weights. K-Mart, Wal Mart, and Target all have a small selection of inexpensive ankle and wrist weights, or you can go to a sports specialty store such as Sports Authority or Big 5 for a better selection. In addition, my websites, beautyandtheyeastbeast.com and ijustblewup.com have a link where you can order attractive, soft Danskin weights, as well as other types of wrist and ankle weights and hand weights. These are all readily available to you on the WWW.

A reminder: you should check with your health care professional prior to embarking on any exercise program.

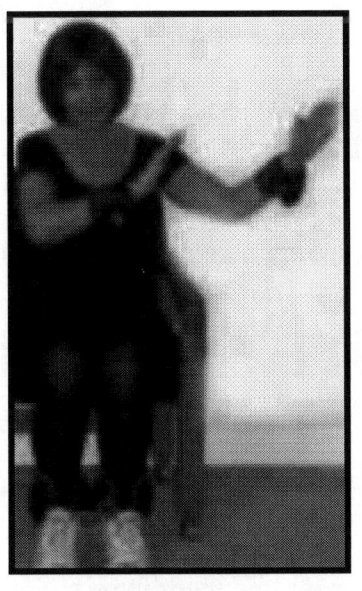

No-exercise is walking around during the day or evening with your wrist and ankle weight on. As soon as you are able, you should move to:

Pre-Exercise Wake-Ups and Metabolism Boosters.

Sit comfortably in a good chair with arms so you can rest your weighed forearms or use the arms to balance yourself when doing leg movements.

Move both of your hands to the left, and then across your torso and to the right, keeping them just below shoulder height.

Doing lazy figure eights in the air will wake up the muscles in your arms and raise your metabolism.

You can hold on to the seat of the chair or the arms, whichever is more comfortable for you.

Do as many different hand movements as you can think of, both with your hands going in the same direction for the movement (e.g. making figure eights in front of you) or in opposite directions (e.g. one up, one down).

I felt silly when I first started these, as a muscle wake up before taking on Godzilla. It's okay to feel silly. Turn on some music, and close your eyes; you will feel so much younger!

This is a tough one for anyone if weighted correctly →

Lift up one knee at a time just about this high. You only want to bring your foot off the floor about 3-4". Keep your foot flat.

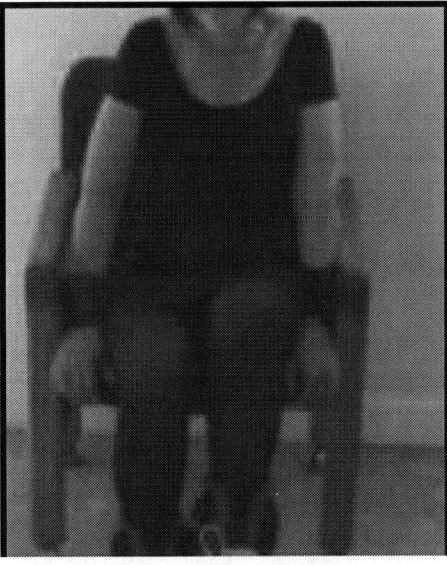

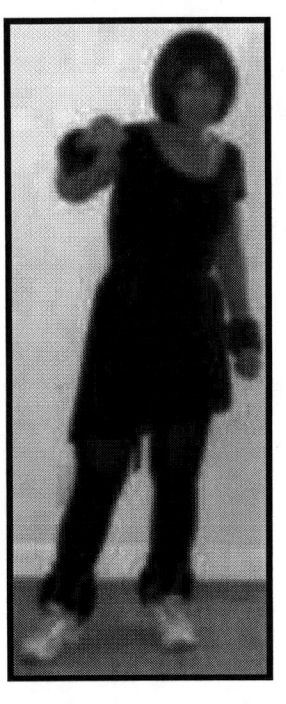

Do you remember doing the Hokey Pokey when you were a kid? As you move around the house with your wrist and ankle weights on, take a minute or two and do the Hokey Pokey as often as you can. Seriously- *You put your <u>right foot</u> in, you put your <u>right foot</u> out, you put your <u>right foot</u> in, and you shake it all about. You do the Hokey Pokey (move in a circle slowly, with your hands in the air above your head, gently waving them) as you turn yourself around, that's what it's all about.* Now repeat this with your left foot, right hand, left hand; then do your whole legs and whole arms. When you get really good, you can take little hops and *put your body in........*

You do the Hokey Pokey and you *<u>turn</u> <u>yourself</u> <u>around</u>....*

That <u>IS</u> what it's all about!

Health Benefits Of Dancing

Calories - During a half hour of dancing you can burn between 200 - 400 calories.
Cardiovascular conditioning - Regular exercise can lead to a slower heart rate, lower blood pressure and improved cholesterol.
Strong bones - Dancing strengthens your weight-bearing bones (tibia, fibula and femur) and can help prevent or slow loss of bone mass (osteoporosis).

Health benefits and risks to dancing depend on how much you put into it. Different types of dance require varying amount of energy.

If you have heart disease or other medical concerns, check with your doctor before taking up dance as a new activity.

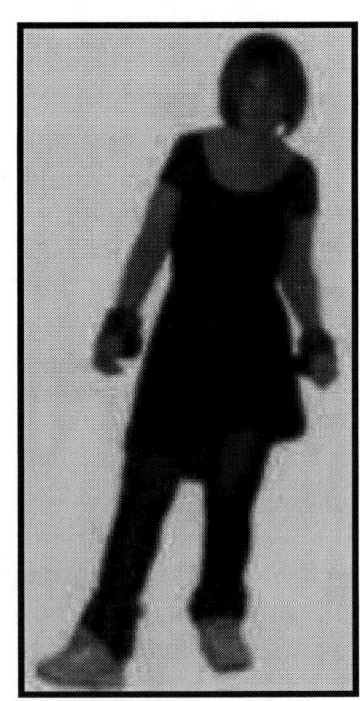

Put on some oldies or some classical or what ever turns you on, and *dance!*

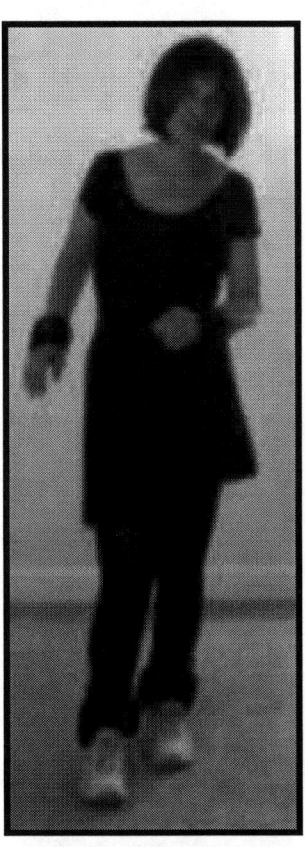

I never exercised until I was 50.

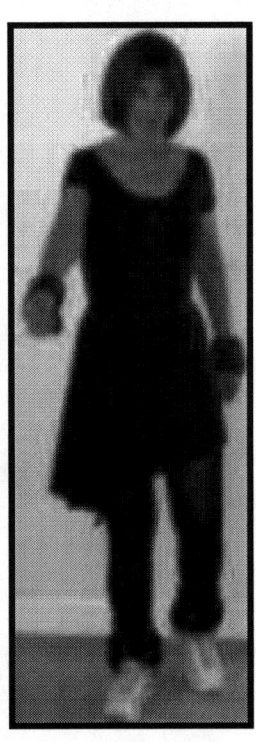

Just dancing around always makes me very self conscious and sometimes embarrassed. But to dance for the camera was actually a great experience. (I was trying to dance very slowly so the pictures would not blur.) It helped to see what I looked like in motion, even if it was a little stifled.

All I was doing here was taking turns moving my arms and legs out and back and sort of rocking a bit to the side. It was like the very easy dance you'd do to rock and roll if you were shy about dancing!

I wear a lot of Danskin because it's well made and very reasonably priced.

Both music and dancing lift the spirit; together they can work miracles!

It is never too late to wake up your muscles and raise your metabolism.

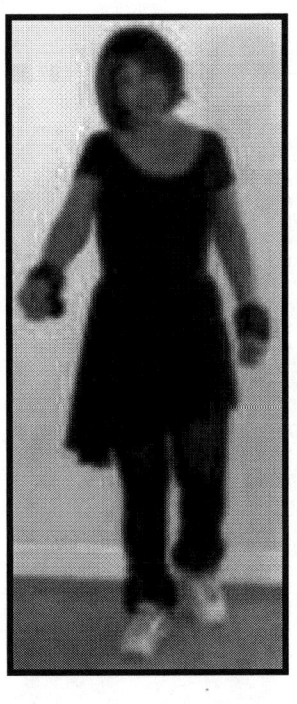

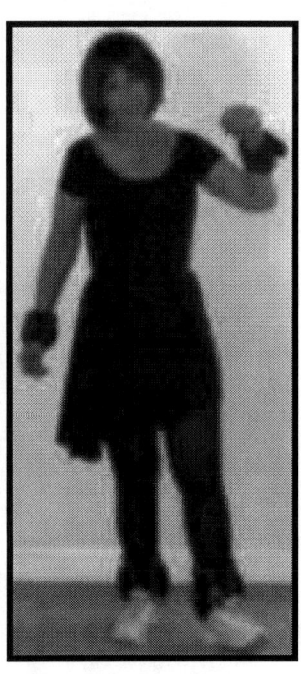

111

Chapter 25
Personal Self-Testing for Yeast and Moulds
(NOTE: Mould is the scientific spelling for mold.)

Yeast in your body is usually commensal (of, relating to, or characterized by a symbiotic relationship in which one species is benefited while the other is unaffected). Broad spectrum antibiotic treatment may be the start of a virulent Yeast/Candida growth as may many other factors, as Yeast is opportunistic and will make a move to take new territory given any chance to do so.

How much is too much?

Unfortunately, the Yeast count in your body is *your* Yeast count and Yeast counts vary from person to person. As there is no benchmark for an acceptable or unacceptable Yeast count in the human body, the only way to know what is going on is to test yourself on an ongoing basis, and create a baseline and ongoing data base to consult to measure your own Yeast count for your own information. Real Yeast testing which will recover a broad spectrum of Yeast is not without cost; it is easier and less expensive to simply presume you have an out of control level of Yeast and consult your physician or health care professional. You may want to bring this book to him/her for review.

Self diagnosis and treatment are growing in popularity; the Candida Self Test (Florida Institute of Mold, Inc.) is a tool for self diagnosis. The Candida Self Test has not been reviewed or approved by the FDA or any recognized medical body. The Candida Self Test will recover Yeast and Yeasts from expelled saliva, skin, and skin folds. The Candida Self Test is not meant to replace your doctor's advice; please consult your health care provider for medical advice.

Do understand that you do *not* need to test yourself. I test myself monthly because I want to know where my Yeast levels are, and often utilize the information I get from the samples to adjust my eating habits or supplement regimen until I see a better result from my self test. But testing is not mandatory, and you should not feel any pressure to test yourself.

If you are like me, and just have to know, you can get information on Yeast self test kits by doing a search on line or by going to my website, personalyeasttestkit.com. At the end of the book there is a coupon for a discount on your first test, should you wish to pursue that.

Chapter 26
When The Yeast Beast Rules

We all know that cookies don't really call to you from the kitchen. However, the Yeast Beast, when it yearns for sugar, makes your body crave it, and when the body craves something, whether it needs it, or because the Yeast Beast is bellowing for it, the mind obliges by remembering where there's a tasty snack to satisfy the urge.

When you hear the call of the Yeast Beast, don't answer.

When the cookies seem to call, and you answer that call, the *Yeast Beast* is in control. It is not *your* weakness; *it is not your fault*. The Yeast Beast works on your body chemically, excreting acetaldehyde, which is a colorless, flammable liquid (C_2H_4O) used to manufacture acetic acid, perfumes, and drugs, also called aldehyde. Acetaldehyde is the toxic compound responsible for most of the maladies of a hangover. There are many other toxins secreted into your system, and the Yeast Beast steals important amino acids, trace minerals, and biotin (which we need to handle stress) from you as well.

The Yeast Beast also wreaks havoc on the psyche. It can make you moody, grouchy, ornery, cantankerous, disagreeable, critical, picky, nit-picky, dissatisfied, agitated, impatient, rude, intolerant, etc. Part of this comes from the effect of the toxins building in your body when you are infested with Candida/Yeast; part of it comes from a (acknowledged or not) deep, and long term unhappiness as a result of long term problems with your weight, an unhappiness (acknowledged or not) which bleeds over into all you do, and affects your relationships at home and at work, as well as out and about amongst strangers.

It is likely to most affect your family. They say *you always hurt the ones you love*; our comfort level within the family seems to breed a tendency to let the Yeast Beast run loose, while in situations with strangers we are more controlled. Don't get too confident there, though; when the Yeast Beast rages, no one is safe.

You will remember my mentioning of the chaos at Starbucks; this kind of behavior and all the other similar behaviors – difficulty at checkout stands, problems with sales people, feeling you have to assert yourself most of the time to get what you need, battles with your children (or your parents, or siblings), general dissatisfaction in your relationships – these are all *Beast Controlled Behaviors*.

If you have been obese for a long time, and are in the latter stages of Candidiasis, you need to understand that these behaviors are woven into the fabric of your personality; when you starve back the Yeast Beast, when you lose the weight, don't expect those behaviors to disappear. And, as your mind has hidden them from you, you will first need to discover them before they can be worked on and removed from your behavior patterns. Also remember that people you have known the longest may be the least able to acknowledge any change in your behavior patterns, and, in some cases, the history of hurt goes so far back there is simply no room in the heart for change.

The Yeast Beast made me do it.

Yeast Beast behavior (we like to call it *Obeastity*) rears its ugly head the hardest when you are tired, hungry, under the influence of alcohol or drugs, in pain, feeling ignored, or emotionally hurting.

Try watching your behavior for a few days. How many times do you immediately respond "no" followed by your justification for disagreeing, with no acknowledgement of what the other person said?

How many times are you "fluffy" (impatient, curt, or snippy) with sales people or on the phone with customer service?

How often do you yell at your children, when all you really want is a quiet cup of coffee and a box of *anything*?

How often do you feel your body just stewing, just grinding on something internally, over and over?

The good news is, once the Yeast Beast is in control, you can take back your nature. The bad news is that you need to learn to recognize the behaviors and substitute more positive behaviors, and that this takes a lot of conscious effort and work. The longer you have been *Beasty*, the harder it is to see/acknowledge these behaviors and the more ingrained the habits are, which make them harder to break.

If you can, find a spouse, life friend, or supportive family member who will sit down with you and honestly list the things about you which they consider to be difficult. Be forewarned: there will be things about you which the person cautiously tells you, but then immediately says they are no big deal, nothing that happens often, certainly a small inconvenience for the value of your friendship: yada, yada.

Ignore this part.

They are trying to be politically correct; they are trying not to hurt your feelings. You need to get them to understand you *know* you have certain behaviors that make you difficult to be around and you want their help in *identifying them for correction*. If you can find someone in your life who will do this for you, you are indeed very lucky, and will most likely come through the process feeling as though you owe that person your life. You may need to hammer in the idea that you really need and want to know for self improvement/self actualization reasons just to get them to be honest; don't forget, while we may be good at criticizing; we probably are not the world's best criticism takers.

Be prepared for hearing the truth about yourself from him/her. Try not to get angry with him/her for being honest; more importantly, try not to get angry with him/her for *not* being honest before, which may be the harder of the two to resist. Know that not many people will offer honest reflection to the Yeast Beast.

Crucial to how we feel is being aware of how we are feeling in the moment. The trick is to realize that we are being emotional in the first place. The earlier we recognize an emotion, the more choices we will have in dealing with it. It's like learning to recognize and stop the spark before the flame leaps. I find that the emotions which are not acknowledged pretty early on get flooded in the drama that goes on around them, and at that point it becomes almost impossible to see the spark; we're already blazing.

A few months ago I was putting away some new makeup, and found myself faced with the issue of not enough space, and a *desperate* decision regarding whether to keep or toss the old makeup, which happened to be from a different company. I came out of the bathroom a few moments later, just laughing out loud at myself, and had to explain to Edward: I had no problem. I was about to make a desperate, difficult, torturous, chaotic situation over the miniscule and innocuous decision of whether to keep or toss some makeup. A year ago the whole issue would have taken an afternoon, at best; I probably would have stewed over what to do and changed my mind eighteen times before making a decision, and I would have involved my husband in my *desperate decision*. What ultimate Beast behavior!!

Look forward to the first time you catch yourself about to be *Beasty* and you stop it in time. It will be one of the most satisfying simple pleasures in your new life.

Glossary

Acetaldehyde – a colorless, flammable liquid, C_2H_4O, used to manufacture acetic acid, perfumes, and drugs; also called aldehyde; acetaldehyde is the compound that produces the symptoms of a hangover

Adipose Tissue – a type of connective tissue that contains stored cellular fat

Adipose Fat – fat stored in connective tissue

Advanced Infirmation – the process of increasingly developing new illness as you age more rapidly than normal due to obesity

Anti-fungal – destroys or inhibits the growth of Fungi

Body Mass Index (BMI) – the most widely accepted measure of obesity, calculated by dividing your weight by the square of your height

Commensal – of, relating to, or characterized by a symbiotic relationship in which one species is benefited while the other is unaffected

Complex carbohydrates – any of a group of organic compounds that includes sugars, starches, celluloses, and gums and serves as a major energy source in the diet of animals. These compounds are produced by photosynthetic plants and contain only carbon, hydrogen, and oxygen, usually in the ratio 1:2:1

Cortisol – a hormone which causes us to crave food

Diet Failure Syndrome – repeated post diet return of weight, usually with additional weight gain, despite the original level of success of the diet

Eat to Live (also see Live to Eat) – days when you feed your body sparsely, giving it sustenance but in small quantities, one food type at a time

Easy greens – this refers to the very low carbohydrate, mostly green, vegetables): Lettuce (all the fun kinds, but not Iceberg), broccoli, cauliflower, spinach, cabbage, cucumbers, bell peppers (preferably red, yellow and orange), asparagus, leek, onion, etc.

Fats – 1-the ester of glycerol and one, two, or three fatty acids. 2- Any of various soft, solid, or semisolid organic compounds constituting the esters of glycerol and fatty acids and their associated organic groups. 3- A mixture of such compounds occurring widely in organic tissue, especially in the adipose tissue of animals and in the seeds, nuts, and fruits of plants. 4- Animal tissue containing such substances. 5- A solidified animal or vegetable oil

Fungi – any of numerous eukaryotic organisms of the kingdom Fungi, which lack Chlorophyll and vascular tissue and range in form from a single cell to a body mass of branched filamentous hyphae that often produce specialized fruiting bodies. The kingdom includes the Yeasts, molds, smuts, and mushrooms

Immune System boosters – supplements offering support to your immune system

Live to Eat (also see Eat to Live) – days you splurge in your eating

Metacarpals – the five cylindrical bones extending from the wrist to the fingers

Metatarsals – the five cylindrical bones extending from the heel to the toes

Micron – measurement; 24,500 microns equal one inch

Morbid Obesity/Gross Obesity (also see Obesity, Unwilling obesity) – morbid obesity is defined by the medical community as more than 100 pounds overweight.

Mucoidal – relating to or resembling mucus; a mucoid substance

Muscle mass – the amount of tissue in your body which is muscle

Naturopathy – naturopathy incorporates a variety of natural approaches (actively through diet, nutrition, supplements, and exercise, and passively through rest, deep breathing, and relaxation) to promote health and well-being on all levels: body, mind and spirit

Nystatin – a prescription drug used to kill off Candida

Obesity (also see Unwilling obesity, Morbid obesity) – very fat or overweight; corpulent; the condition of being obese; increased body weight caused by excessive accumulation of fat

Obeastity – the psychological behaviors exhibited when affected by the Yeast Beast

Optimum Recovery – mold terminology for gathering from an area to be tested all of the various spores in an area and propagating in a way that allows for all the species that are present to grow

Overweight – weighing more than the limit for your height and age on standard height and weight charts

Phasing – changing from one form to another

Probiotic – general term for a substance that promotes the growth of microorganisms

Proteins – any of a group of complex organic macromolecules that contain carbon, hydrogen, oxygen, nitrogen, and usually sulfur and are composed of one or more chains of amino acids. Proteins are fundamental components of all living cells and include many substances, such as enzymes, hormones, and antibodies which are necessary for the proper functioning of an organism. They are essential in the diet of animals for the growth and repair of tissue and can be obtained from foods such as meat, fish, eggs, milk, and legumes

Self-subjugation – to make one's self subservient; enslaved

Serendipity – the faculty of making fortunate discoveries by accident

Single Species Recovery – propagating in a way that limits the species present which will grow in a medium by altering the composition of the medium to rule out species not specifically being sought

Sugar – a sweet crystalline or powdered substance, white when pure, consisting of sucrose obtained mainly from sugar cane and sugar beets and used in many foods, drinks, and medicines to improve their taste; any of a class of water-soluble crystalline carbohydrates, including sucrose and lactose, having a characteristically sweet taste and classified as monosaccharides, disaccharides, and trisaccharides.

Unwilling obesity – existing in a state of obesity despite one's efforts to lose weight

Visceral fat – fat that accumulates around the organs

Viscous – having relatively high resistance to flow; of a glutinous nature or consistency; sticky; thick; adhesive

Wrist Weights – weighted bands made to wear on your wrist; usually held on by Velcro straps

Yeast – any of various unicellular Fungi reproducing by budding, form ascospores and are capable of fermenting carbohydrates

Yeast Beast – popular term for Yeast overgrowth

Yo-Yo dieting – a series of successful diets which result in post diet weight return; often more weight is gained after the diet than lost on the diet

About the Author

Francine Hemway earned a Bachelor's Degree from Sonoma State University in English, and a Master's Degree from San Diego State University in Educational Administration. She is a retired elementary and secondary teacher and public school administrator. She holds California Credentials for School Administration, Elementary Education, Secondary Education English, Secondary Education Life Science, Secondary Education Consumer Education, Secondary Education Psychology, and Community College English/ESL (English as a Second Language), an Arizona State School Principal's Certificate, and is a licensed Obesity Counselor. She currently owns and operates the Florida Institute of Mold, where she heads the Yeast Research Division of the Optimum Recovery Laboratory, and the Publications Division, though she keeps active in the Mold Inspection and Remediation Division as a licensed mold inspector. A victim the Yeast Beast and the *Curse of the Yeast Beast*, she was overweight from childhood and morbidly obese for over a decade. She battled the Yeast Beast, lost 180 pounds, which she has kept off for over five years, conquered the Curse of the Yeast Beast, and has successfully renovated the battleground, both physically and psychologically.

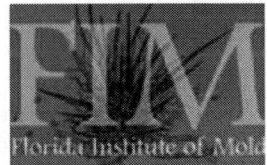

Florida Institute of Mold Websites

Below is a listing of all of the FIM websites for your information and reference. To make it easier to read, the list is presented as site titles, not URL's (WWW addresses).

Each website title should be used in the form of a **.com** with no spaces or capitals.

Example: <u>Allergen Fight Back</u> website address is: <u>allergenfightback.com</u>

Allergen Fight Back
Beauty and the Yeast Beast
Best Mold Test Kit
Bye Bye Yeast
Bye Bye Yeast Beast
Candida Buster
Candida Candida
Candida Recovery Laboratories
Candida spp
Candida Treatment Program
Candida Weight Loss
Certified Yeast Inspector
Doctor Yeast
End the Obesity
Euclidian Magniscopy
Fat to Fairy Tale
Florida Institute of Mold
Florida Institute of Yeast
I Just Blew Up
Mold Professor
Modern Mold Test Kit

NoMo Yo-Yo dieting
Obese Recovery
Obesity Rehab
One Stop Candida Shop
Personal Yeast Test Kit
Phasing Center
Scientific Mold Test Kit
Yeast Across America
Yeast Beast Control
Yeast Inspection
Yeast Inspector
Yeast Med
Yeast Professor
Yeast Remediation
Yeast Remediator
Yeast Technologies
Yeast Test Kit
Yeast Testing
Yeast Treatment Program
Yeast Treatment Center

Save $5.00
on your first bottle of
Grapefruit Seed Extract

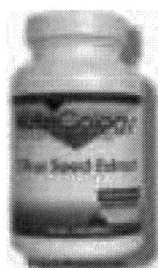

Grapefruit Seed Extract Regularly $23.00

Free Shipping + Handling
Send your check for $18.00 and the completed form below to:

Florida Institute of Mold
4801 Linton Blvd. #11A
PMB 612
Delray Beach FL 33445
Attn: Beauty

Form Has Name Address

Give *Beauty and the Yeast Beast*
To Someone special and
Save $5.00

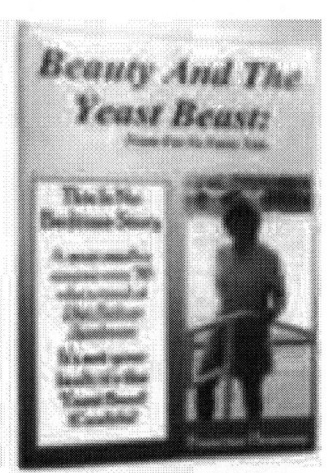

Beauty and the Yeast Beast: From Fat to Fairy Tale
Regularly $39.95
Free Shipping and Handling
Send your check for $34.95 and the completed form below to:

Florida Institute of Mold
4801 Linton Blvd. #11A
PMB 612
Delray Beach FL 33445
Attn: Beauty

===

NAME: _____

ADDRESS: _____

CITY: _____ STATE: _____ ZIP: _____

e-mail (optional): _____

Save $20.00 on
Fight Back Vaporizing Air Cleanser

<u>Asthma Allergy Sinusitis and Yeast Suffers *Fight Back!*</u>
Fungal aeroallergens are known to exasperate Asthma Allergy and Sinusitis. You now have an effective way to Fight Back and gain control of the air in your home and office.

**Regularly
4/$99.00**

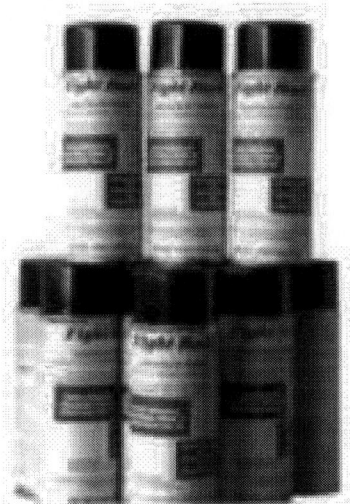

*<u>Fight Back Gets
Yeast
out of the Air</u>*

Yeast in your bedroom? Clean the air the safe and effective way with *Fight Back* today and sleep well tonight.

**For more information:
Call 561.577.7202**
allergenfightback.com

Non Flammable Non Toxic

Send your check for $85.00 ($79.00 + 6.00 S&H) and the completed form below to:

Florida Institute of Mold
4801 Linton Blvd. #11A
PMB 612
Delray Beach FL 33445
Attn: Beauty

===

NAME: _____

ADDRESS: _____

CITY: _____ STATE: _____ ZIP: _____

e-mail (optional): _____

Save 20%
On Your First
Personal Yeast Test Kit

FOR A THOROUGH
EXPLANATION OF THE
CONTENTS AND
PROCEDURES OF THE
YEAST TEST KIT, PLEASE
GO TO OUR WEBSITE,

personalyeasttestkit.com

Personal Yeast Test Kit Regularly $89.95
Kit Is A 3 Sample Series

Send your check for $77.00 ($71.50 + $5.50 S&H)
and the completed form below to:

Florida Institute of Mold
4801 Linton Blvd. #11A
PMB 612
Delray Beach FL 33445
Attn: Beauty

NAME: _____

ADDRESS: _____

CITY: _____ STATE: _____ ZIP: _____

e-mail (optional): _____

Daily Journal

How To Use This Journal

Numerous books have been written about the benefits to journaling and how to journal. Later, you may wish to investigate journal writing further. For the purposes of this journal, the pages are set up simply with very little structure; this allows you the freedom to structure your entries to suit your individuality.

Do put the date on each page. Entering your weight is optional; if putting the numbers in print is traumatic for you, don't do it at first. Some people like to weight themselves every day, some once a week. All kind of advice is available on this: how often to weigh yourself, and when, and under what conditions, and most of it is conflicting. Do what works for you.

I believe that one should weight one's self daily, naked or in a night gown or whatever you chose, at about the same time of day. I weigh myself in the morning after I've had my coffee. It doesn't matter when you weigh yourself, but it does matter that you weigh yourself about the same time every day. When I did Weight Watchers, I would always go to meetings first and eat dinner afterwards; what can I say, I was 14 and thought that not eating first made a difference. When you weigh yourself daily, you need to keep a mental average in your head, as not only do daily weights fluctuate, but weights taken at different times of the day do as well. I find I get a more accurate picture – and an earlier wake up call if I'm going too far – when I keep that in my head rather than take the one measurement once a week.

Strengths and weaknesses are vague categories you can utilize to record where you're feeling successful and where you're feeling like you are not doing as well. Strengths are things like passed up dessert, protein spread evenly throughout the day, survived Aunt Tillie's 80th birthday party without sharing her cake; you can use this to record whatever information will be helpful to you to keep your resolve strong, and to acknowledge your successes.

Weaknesses can be recordings of slips – oops: that piece of cheesecake just got me; it can be times of the day you notice you have more difficulty. It can record thoughts about yourself, others, the program, etc. The list of uses for the journal is endless and is meant to be personalized. Make this journal yours; make it work for you. You will be directed throughout the program to review your journal for information; the more you put into your journal, the more you will get from it later.

Affirmations are statements you repeat to yourself until they become unconscious thoughts. Throughout the journal are scattered suggested affirmations; they appear in italics: *I will not let the Yeast Beast win today.* We internal chatter all the time. Direct this chatter into supportive messages to yourself. This may seen forced at first, but it becomes easier.

Saying something positive to yourself in front of the mirror five or six times each morning will re-train your thought pattern about your body and weight loss. Several affirmations are given in the quotes at the end of various journal pages. You can use these, or make up your own. Affirmations are not given for every day, but do try to spend five minutes in the mirror each morning repeating these and other phrases to yourself – out loud if you can. (Go ahead; run the water).

One note about affirmations: the mind does not know what is true and what is not, and it believes what you tell it. If you repeat to yourself mentally that you are fat and it's never going to get any better, your mind will internalize this information and actually work to make it so. If you feed your mind one-liners about getting thin, getting healthy, not needing so overeat, etc. your mind will work to make those things reality.

Some of my favorites are *I don't need much food at a time to be satisfied. I graze throughout the day because my body performs optimally on small amounts ingested frequently. The Yeast Beast stole much of my life; I am in charge of my life now, not the Beast.* My all time favorite and the hardest one sometimes, is *I deserve to be healthy and fit.* Don't be afraid to make up your own; don't be afraid to make them big statements; when I was at 165 pounds, I started telling myself, *I only weighted 135 and it is easy to choose food types and quantities to maintain that weight.* Of course, I still weighted 160. But I kept saying it, and eventually did weigh 135.

You might make note of any compliments you receive, thoughts about yourself that you noticed (positive and negative), and reactions to various situations. Experiment with what you write, and don't worry if it seems silly or boring. What you write today will provide insight tomorrow, no matter how unimpressive the information seems on the day written. Let your mind flow when you journal.

Try to take ten to twenty minutes for yourself daily in a quiet place to do this journaling. If you have kids, you can get them composition books and let them do their own journals with you; it will entertain them, make them feel like they're doing what you're doing, and give them practice in their writing skills. Who knows – you may have a budding writer in the family!

A word about photos: no one hated having photos taken more than I did. (I still am not thrilled by it and tend to freeze up when confronted with a camera.) I am in almost no family pictures, particularly since I learned about *taking* pictures: the person <u>with</u> the camera is safe <u>from</u> the camera. I became the family photo historian out of self protection.

Take a before picture now. Wear something that fits you now, and don't choose that one dress or pants set that makes you look slimmer; take a hard straight on shot with no tummy holding and no forced posturing. Let the real you get put on film. I kept my before picture safe, but well hidden, for years.

Try to get someone to take your picture from front, back and side. We may not *see* what the mirror reflects, but we surely don't see what others see behind us!

Take new photos whenever you see noticeable differences; I suggest you put the date on each picture, and, if you're not shy about it, the current weight. Make up an alphabet code if you have to, or simply write minus 3 (whatever number) pounds; you can always figure it out from that later! Keep the photos with your journal (you can glue an envelope inside the back cover). These will be of great help when resolve wanes, or on days the Yeast Beast is bellowing so loudly you're ready to empty the shelves at Dunkin donuts to quiet it!

Make this your journal; no one ever need see it. Do it for *you*.

Daily Journal – Day 1

Date:
Weight:
Strengths:
Weaknesses:
Notes (how you felt, what influenced food choices, exercise/weights time, etc.):

Today you declare war; welcome to Yeast Beast boot camp.
Remember, you can do anything for 24 hours.

Daily Journal – Day 2

Date:
Weight:
Strengths:
Weaknesses:
Notes (how you felt, what influenced food choices, exercise/weights time, etc.):

You've got the Beast's attention now! Don't let its demands for sugar and flour get you off track. If you get _Beasty_, take a few deep breaths. Remind yourself you're at war.

Daily Journal – Day 3

Date:
Weight:
Strengths:
Weaknesses:
Notes (how you felt, what influenced food choices, exercise/weights time, etc.):

You're still here; great! Today should be the last hard day; if you've stayed on protein and salad, you should notice your desire for Yeast Beast food decreasing, and your ability to decline it increasing.

Daily Journal – Day 4

Date:	
Weight:	
Strengths:	
Weaknesses:	

Notes (how you felt, what influenced food choices, exercise/weights time, etc.):

I will not let the Yeast Beast win today. We internal chatter all the time. Direct this chatter to supportive affirmations, things you repeat to yourself until they become unconscious thoughts.

Daily Journal – Day 5

Date:	
Weight:	
Strengths:	
Weaknesses:	
Notes (how you felt, what influenced food choices, exercise/weights time, etc.):	

Take your anti-fungals and probiotics when you first get up; don't eat anything for 30 minutes, but do eat a good protein breakfast as soon as you can after that.

Daily Journal – Day 6

Date:
Weight:
Strengths:
Weaknesses:
Notes (how you felt, what influenced food choices, exercise/weights time, etc.):

Let's talk about movement. Are you exercising or wearing hand and ankle weights? Fidget whenever you can; it helps burn calories and raise metabolism.

Daily Journal – Day 7

Date:
Weight:
Strengths:
Weaknesses:
Notes (how you felt, what influenced food choices, exercise/weights time, etc.):

You've made it half way through Phase One! Look back on your journal; pay attention to where you focused your attention in what you chose to write. What did you learn from your writing? What other information would you like to include for future benefit?

Daily Journal – Day 8

Date:
Weight:
Strengths:
Weaknesses:
Notes (how you felt, what influenced food choices, exercise/weights time, etc.):

You can overeat carbs until the cows come home, but the body says stop when its had enough protein. Eat all the protein you can, and allow yourself butter and mayo and cheese. You may be cutting them out later when you switch diets!

Daily Journal – Day 9

Date:
Weight:
Strengths:
Weaknesses:
Notes (how you felt, what influenced food choices, exercise/weights time, etc.):

Have you taken your picture? *The Yeast Beast has controlled me long enough; now I am gaining control over the Yeast Beast.*

Daily Journal – Day 10

Date:	
Weight:	
Strengths:	
Weaknesses:	

Notes (how you felt, what influenced food choices, exercise/weights time, etc.):

String cheese individually packed is a lifesaver. Any restaurant can get you eggs most any way you want them.

Daily Journal – Day 10

Date:	
Weight:	
Strengths:	
Weaknesses:	

Notes (how you felt, what influenced food choices, exercise/weights time, etc.):

The Yeast Beast has ruined how many years of your life with unwanted weight gain, in fact unwilling obesity? Enough – stay in control of the Yeast Beast today. *I will not let the Yeast Beast beat me.*

Daily Journal – Day 11

Date:
Weight:
Strengths:
Weaknesses:
Notes (how you felt, what influenced food choices, exercise/weights time, etc.):

I lost the weight without Gastrointestinal bypass or Liposuction. Control the Yeast Beast today and the weight will go away. You're almost done with Phase One; keep up the great work, and don't forget to acknowledge yourself!

Daily Journal – Day 12

Date:	
Weight:	
Strengths:	
Weaknesses:	

Notes (how you felt, what influenced food choices, exercise/weights time, etc.):

You cannot kill the Yeast Beast, but you can punish the Yeast Beast and reduce its numbers by eating right and moving.
Today I will starve and punish the Yeast Beast.

Daily Journal – Day 13

Date:
Weight:
Strengths:
Weaknesses:
Notes (how you felt, what influenced food choices, exercise/weights time, etc.):

The Yeast Beast never sleeps; never let your guard down; punish the Yeast Beast by feeding your body properly. Boot camp is almost over; you've got the Beast on the run.

Daily Journal – Day 14

Date:	
Weight:	
Strengths:	
Weaknesses:	

Notes (how you felt, what influenced food choices, exercise/weights time, etc.):

The Yeast Beast loves sugar and flour. Starve the Yeast Beast today. Review the diet today, reminding yourself of the new options available to you starting tomorrow. Start planning now so that tomorrow goes as planned.

Daily Journal – Day 15

| Date: |
| Weight: |
| Strengths: |
| |
| |
| |
| Weaknesses: |
| |
| |
| |
| Notes (how you felt, what influenced food choices, exercise/weights time, etc.): |
| |
| |
| |
| |
| |
| |
| |
| |
| |
| |
| |
| |
| |
| |
| |
| |
| |
| |
| |
| |

Time to raise the ante on exercise/no exercise just a bit. Start working longer, and work towards extending your range of motion; don't try to raise both on the same day.

Daily Journal – Day 16

Date:
Weight:
Strengths:
Weaknesses:
Notes (how you felt, what influenced food choices, exercise/weights time, etc.):

The Yeast Beast hates protein; have a steak. *The Yeast Beast used to control me; today I am in control of the Beast.*

Daily Journal – Day 17

Date:	
Weight:	
Strengths:	
Weaknesses:	

Notes (how you felt, what influenced food choices, exercise/weights time, etc.):

The Yeast Beast makes you grow old and weak. *Old age ain't for sissies* **(Bette Davis) didn't even** <u>*consider*</u> **obese old age.**

Daily Journal – Day 18

Date:
Weight:
Strengths:
Weaknesses:
Notes (how you felt, what influenced food choices, exercise/weights time, etc.):

How are you doing with new foods? If you feel that new energy waning just a bit, make sure you're not introducing too much too soon.

Daily Journal – Day 19

Date:	
Weight:	
Strengths:	

Weaknesses:

Notes (how you felt, what influenced food choices, exercise/weights time, etc.):

Whose body is it, yours or the Yeast Beast's? Fight the Yeast Beast; get control.

Daily Journal – Day 20

Date:
Weight:
Strengths:
Weaknesses:
Notes (how you felt, what influenced food choices, exercise/weights time, etc.):

Listen to your body. It will tell you when you are hungry, and, if you listen carefully it will tell you what it needs. Don't be fooled by calls for goodies; that's the Beast, not your body.

Daily Journal – Day 21

Date:	
Weight:	
Strengths:	
Weaknesses:	

Notes (how you felt, what influenced food choices, exercise/weights time, etc.):

Punish the Yeast Beast today; eat what is good for you and bad for the Yeast Beast. Win today in the Yeast Beast fight. You're half way through Phase Two. Look back over your journal. How far you've come; how far you can go!

Daily Journal – Day 22

Date:	
Weight:	
Strengths:	
Weaknesses:	

Notes (how you felt, what influenced food choices, exercise/weights time, etc.):

Focus on the Yeast Beast inside you and get control. The war is won one battle at a time, one right choice at a time. It's not your will power; it's a test of wills against the Beast.

Daily Journal – Day 23

Date:	
Weight:	
Strengths:	
Weaknesses:	

Notes (how you felt, what influenced food choices, exercise/weights time, etc.):

Now that you know what has been causing your weight gain, you're getting control and will live a life without the Yeast Beast inside you. *The Beast has stolen from me: stolen my looks, stolen opportunities. The Beast will steal from me mo more.*

Daily Journal – Day 24

Date:	
Weight:	
Strengths:	
Weaknesses:	
Notes (how you felt, what influenced food choices, exercise/weights time, etc.):	

The Yeast Beast want a bigger you and wants you to be sedentary and eat pastry.

Daily Journal – Day 25

Date:	
Weight:	
Strengths:	

Weaknesses:

Notes (how you felt, what influenced food choices, exercise/weights time, etc.):

Take your anti-fungals and probiotics; get the Yeast Beast.

Daily Journal – Day 26

Date:	
Weight:	
Strengths:	
Weaknesses:	

Notes (how you felt, what influenced food choices, exercise/weights time, etc.):

Spend ten full minutes in the mirror when you get dressed or undressed. Lock the door if you need to, but try to unlock your blocked vision. This takes lots of practice.

Daily Journal – Day 27

Date:	
Weight:	
Strengths:	
Weaknesses:	

Notes (how you felt, what influenced food choices, exercise/weights time, etc.):

This is the last day of Phase Two; review the Phase Three of the diet in the book. This involves serious thought before tomorrow! Remember, once you move to another diet, your unlimited amounts of protein (of everything) must be portion controlled.

Daily Journal – Day 28

Date:
Weight:
Strengths:
Weaknesses:
Notes (how you felt, what influenced food choices, exercise/weights time, etc.):

Congratulations: you complete Phase Two today! The Yeast Beast hates exercise; the more you move the more you flush your system of the Yeast Beast. Time to step up your exercise/no exercise routine.

Daily Journal – Day 29

Date:
Weight:
Strengths:
Weaknesses:
Notes (how you felt, what influenced food choices, exercise/weights time, etc.):

Today could be your day to switch anti-fungals and hit the Beast with a new punch; get the Beast. Keep the Beast off guard; switch your anti-fungals every 3-4 weeks.

Daily Journal – Day 30

Date:
Weight:
Strengths:
Weaknesses:
Notes (how you felt, what influenced food choices, exercise/weights time, etc.):

The Yeast Beast thinks you are its home. The Yeast Beast wants you to eat what *it* wants, and for you to gain as much weight as possible; starve the Yeast Beast today. *I am winning this war against the Beast.*

Daily Journal – Day 31

Date:
Weight:
Strengths:
Weaknesses:
Notes (how you felt, what influenced food choices, exercise/weights time, etc.):

Define for yourself who you can count on for support in your quest to conquer the Beast. Ask for that help.

Daily Journal – Day 32

Date:	
Weight:	
Strengths:	
Weaknesses:	
Notes (how you felt, what influenced food choices, exercise/weights time, etc.):	

The Yeast Beast is relentless: morning, noon, and night the Beast is ever vigilant. Every late night snack desire is the Beast. *I know when I'm hungry and when the Beast is bellowing.*

Daily Journal – Day 33

Date:	
Weight:	
Strengths:	
Weaknesses:	

Notes (how you felt, what influenced food choices, exercise/weights time, etc.):

As time goes on it gets easier to fight the Yeast Beast. How are you feeling with the new diet? Are you retaining energy? Are you managing portion control? Step up your range of motion or the length of your workout. If you've been doing no

exercise, it's time to try some. Try walking ten minutes a day for now; do more as you can. Don't forget your weights!

Daily Journal – Day 34

Date:
Weight:
Strengths:
Weaknesses:
Notes (how you felt, what influenced food choices, exercise/weights time, etc.):

Yeast Beast has been working on you for quite a while and it is time to get even. The Yeast Beast made you heavy; now make the Yeast Beast small. *I am in a war with the Yeast Beast. My life depends on winning this war.*

Daily Journal – Day 35

Date:
Weight:
Strengths:
Weaknesses:
Notes (how you felt, what influenced food choices, exercise/weights time, etc.):

You're halfway through Phase Three. This is a great time to review your journal. It's also time to take another photograph.

Daily Journal – Day 36

Date:
Weight:
Strengths:
Weaknesses:
Notes (how you felt, what influenced food choices, exercise/weights time, etc.):

The Yeast Beast likes it when you eat until you feel full and you are. An overstuffed stomach makes more room for the Beast to grow. *It just doesn't take that much to fill me up any more. I stop every two or three bites to see how full I am so I don't overeat.*

Daily Journal – Day 37

Date:
Weight:
Strengths:
Weaknesses:
Notes (how you felt, what influenced food choices, exercise/weights time, etc.):

Shrink your stomach and shrink Yeast Beast territory.

Daily Journal – Day 38

Date:
Weight:
Strengths:
Weaknesses:
Notes (how you felt, what influenced food choices, exercise/weights time, etc.):

Today is the easiest day of my life to fight the Yeast Beast. *I am winning this war.*

Daily Journal – Day 39

Date:
Weight:
Strengths:
Weaknesses:
Notes (how you felt, what influenced food choices, exercise/weights time, etc.):

Fight the Yeast Beast today and grow old thin and limber. Extra efforts in the Yeast Beast fight today give you better days, and more of them, in the future.

Daily Journal – Day 40

Date:
Weight:
Strengths:
Weaknesses:
Notes (how you felt, what influenced food choices, exercise/weights time, etc.):

Walking with wrist and ankle weight is the biggest step in comfortable exercise there is; start as soon as possible. Try an exercise video, dance to your favorite music, or just lower the tension bar all the way on the vacuum! *I add/increase exercise in my life because I am banking health for my future.*

Daily Journal – Day 41

Date:	
Weight:	
Strengths:	

Weaknesses:

Notes (how you felt, what influenced food choices, exercise/weights time, etc.):

I push old age and disease away as I control the Beast today. **Tomorrow you move to the diet of your choice. If you are still comfortable with the Phase Three diet, you are welcome to stay there a while longer. Be sure your new diet is Beast proofed.**

Daily Journal – Day 42

Date:
Weight:
Strengths:
Weaknesses:
Notes (how you felt, what influenced food choices, exercise/weights time, etc.):

Have you been spending time with the mirror? Spend five minutes today looking at yourself in the mirror, privately. Note and/or record your observations, and your emotions. Don't be critical; just work on seeing what is being reflected.

Daily Journal – Day 43

Date:
Weight:
Strengths:
Weaknesses:
Notes (how you felt, what influenced food choices, exercise/weights time, etc.):

Controlling the Yeast Beast today means you are in control of your life tomorrow. Pull out the photos from the start of the program. Reward yourself with something small and personal, something non-food.

Daily Journal – Day 44

Date:
Weight:
Strengths:
Weaknesses:
Notes (how you felt, what influenced food choices, exercise/weights time, etc.):

You do not want to grow old obese; it is a miserable existence. Every day you stay on this program you are banking for future health, and the ability to enjoy your retirement years.

Daily Journal – Day 45

Date:
Weight:
Strengths:
Weaknesses:
Notes (how you felt, what influenced food choices, exercise/weights time, etc.):

Time to reflect, take pictures, journey back through your
journal and photos; by now you surely can see a different you,
and can feel what you feel like when the
Beast is not controlling you.

Daily Journal – Day 46

Date:	
Weight:	
Strengths:	
Weaknesses:	

Notes (how you felt, what influenced food choices, exercise/weights time, etc.):

Being overweight slows down your career and earning power; stop being cheated. Get control of the weight today and starve the Yeast Beast today.

Daily Journal – Day 47

Date:
Weight:
Strengths:
Weaknesses:
Notes (how you felt, what influenced food choices, exercise/weights time, etc.):

Staying healthy means controlling the Yeast Beast. The number of ailments attributed to being overweight is numerous. *I am working today to be healthy for tomorrow.*

Daily Journal – Day 48

Date:
Weight:
Strengths:
Weaknesses:
Notes (how you felt, what influenced food choices, exercise/weights time, etc.):

The Yeast Beast is an organism that has the basic drives of all living organisms, including a nice place to live and that means a bigger you; starve the Yeast Beast and get a smaller you.

Daily Journal – Day 49

Date:
Weight:
Strengths:
Weaknesses:
Notes (how you felt, what influenced food choices, exercise/weights time, etc.):

Being overweight directly affects the quality of your life. Your health as you grow older becomes more important in defining what you are able to do and enjoy. Starve the Yeast Beast now and live better as you get older.

Daily Journal – Day 50

Date:
Weight:
Strengths:
Weaknesses:
Notes (how you felt, what influenced food choices, exercise/weights time, etc.):

Deep breathing should be a part of your get healthy routine. As you concentrate on your breathing, do an affirmation that helps you focus on your success and your strength. You are a warrior. *I am a warrior.*

Daily Journal – Day 51

Date:
Weight:
Strengths:
Weaknesses:
Notes (how you felt, what influenced food choices, exercise/weights time, etc.):

Watch whatever makes you laugh hard. Laugh a lot and laugh hard for an hour a day; you will feel better and so will your insides.

Daily Journal – Day 52

Date:
Weight:
Strengths:
Weaknesses:
Notes (how you felt, what influenced food choices, exercise/weights time, etc.):

Invest the time and energy into yourself; take your anti-fungals and at least wear wrist weights to get the blood flowing. *My body wants to work, and needs to work. I am helping it get strong so it will work optimally for me.*

Daily Journal – Day 53

Date:
Weight:
Strengths:
Weaknesses:
Notes (how you felt, what influenced food choices, exercise/weights time, etc.):

You are getting stronger; keep the pressure on the Yeast Beast and work out extra. An extra 10 minutes of walking with weights wrist and ankle really hurts the Yeast Beast. Breathe deeply as you walk.

Daily Journal – Day 54

Date:	
Weight:	
Strengths:	

Weaknesses:

Notes (how you felt, what influenced food choices, exercise/weights time, etc.):

Fighting the Yeast Beast is a way of life; the Yeast Beast will never give up and neither should you.

Daily Journal – Day 55

Date:
Weight:
Strengths:
Weaknesses:
Notes (how you felt, what influenced food choices, exercise/weights time, etc.):

Dropping the weight: you've done it before. This time the weight will stay gone because you are learning how to control the Yeast Beast.

Daily Journal – Day 56

Date:
Weight:
Strengths:
Weaknesses:
Notes (how you felt, what influenced food choices, exercise/weights time, etc.):

Vitamins are needed if you are very heavy and have had a lot of baked goods in your diet. A diet of baked goods will leave you malnourished.

Daily Journal – Day 57

Date:
Weight:
Strengths:
Weaknesses:
Notes (how you felt, what influenced food choices, exercise/weights time, etc.):

Test the air in your bedroom. Are you breathing airborne Yeast in your sleep? You need to clean up the Yeast in your home. You might want to check out Allergen Fight Back Air Cleanser at <u>allergenfightback.com</u>

Daily Journal – Day 58

Date:	
Weight:	
Strengths:	
Weaknesses:	

Notes (how you felt, what influenced food choices, exercise/weights time, etc.):

This day is a most important day to control the Yeast Beast as is every day of your life because the Yeast Beast wants you to eat sugar and flour and starch and get as big as possible. *I am in control of me; I am no longer a slave to the Beast.*

Daily Journal – Day 59

Date:
Weight:
Strengths:
Weaknesses:
Notes (how you felt, what influenced food choices, exercise/weights time, etc.):

Fighting the Yeast Beast means taking your anti-fungals and probiotics faithfully. After your initial 90-120 day Beast battle is over, you should take probiotics continually and anti-fungals for 30 days every three months.

Daily Journal – Day 60

Date:
Weight:
Strengths:
Weaknesses:
Notes (how you felt, what influenced food choices, exercise/weights time, etc.):

You're at the halfway point of the Yeast control program: congratulations! Stick with the program; reclaim your life from the Yeast Beast.

Daily Journal – Day 61

Date:	
Weight:	
Strengths:	
Weaknesses:	

Notes (how you felt, what influenced food choices, exercise/weights time, etc.):

Always think before you eat: who you are eating for, you or the Yeast Beast? You have to beat the Yeast Beast every day.

Daily Journal – Day 62

Date:	
Weight:	
Strengths:	

Weaknesses:

Notes (how you felt, what influenced food choices, exercise/weights time, etc.):

When you move and get your blood flowing let yourself get a little hungry; then have a small amount of cold protein and wait ten minutes. Your hunger will abate for quite a while.

Daily Journal – Day 63

Date:
Weight:
Strengths:
Weaknesses:
Notes (how you felt, what influenced food choices, exercise/weights time, etc.):

Stretching carefully every day is a great way to increase blood circulation and help cleanse your system. If you're working out, do some stretching before and after your workout. Take lessons from the cat, one of God's most limber creatures. It never gets up without stretching, and it naps when its tired.

Daily Journal – Day 64

Date:	
Weight:	
Strengths:	

Weaknesses:

Notes (how you felt, what influenced food choices, exercise/weights time, etc.):

Beating back the Beast you must decide how much work you are willing to do for your later life health. Getting slim and staying slender is the best thing you can do to protect yourself from falls. *I am winning the battle with the Beast by making sound choices about food and movement.*

Daily Journal – Day 65

Date:
Weight:
Strengths:
Weaknesses:
Notes (how you felt, what influenced food choices, exercise/weights time, etc.):

Not eating that donut hurts the Yeast Beast more than it hurts you. *The Beast hurt me for (# years); <u>no more</u>. The more I hurt the Beast, the healthier I become.*

Daily Journal – Day 66

Date:	
Weight:	
Strengths:	

Weaknesses:

Notes (how you felt, what influenced food choices, exercise/weights time, etc.):

We are informationally rich, mechanically strong and biologically weak. We need to be as strong as possible to face old age and retirement.

Daily Journal – Day 67

| Date: |
| Weight: |
| Strengths: |

Weaknesses:

Notes (how you felt, what influenced food choices, exercise/weights time, etc.):

Eat to live today. To fight the Yeast Beast you must not feed the Yeast Beast. *I choose what I eat to serve my body today. I will eat for pleasure less frequently.*

Daily Journal – Day 68

Date:	
Weight:	
Strengths:	
Weaknesses:	

Notes (how you felt, what influenced food choices, exercise/weights time, etc.):

You have learned that the Yeast Beast is not happy that you are not feeding it. You should have dropped a significant amount of weight by this time as you have in all you other diet attempts; now is the day to really get control of the Yeast Beast.

Daily Journal – Day 69

Date:	
Weight:	
Strengths:	
Weaknesses:	

Notes (how you felt, what influenced food choices, exercise/weights time, etc.):

This is the danger zone in the past; all yo-yo dieters start to gain about this period of time after some successful weight loss. Keep controlling the Yeast Beast; watch those Yeast foods!

Daily Journal – Day 70

Date:
Weight:
Strengths:
Weaknesses:
Notes (how you felt, what influenced food choices, exercise/weights time, etc.):

A change of diet may be in order at this time but take your anti-fungals and put some extra effort into metabolic stimulation. Laugh, deep breaths, or stretch for an extra 15 minutes and get the Yeast Beast.

Daily Journal – Day 71

Date:
Weight:
Strengths:
Weaknesses:
Notes (how you felt, what influenced food choices, exercise/weights time, etc.):

The Yeast Beast expects you to lose at first; at this point in your program, the Yeast Beast expects you to go back to Danish. Stick to your chosen program today. *I am not only what I eat; more importantly, I am what I don't eat.*

Daily Journal – Day 72

Date:
Weight:
Strengths:
Weaknesses:
Notes (how you felt, what influenced food choices, exercise/weights time, etc.):

Inside of you the Yeast Beast is very unhappy: 71 days of no sugar or flour. Show the Beast who is in control; you are over half way there. *I am in control.*

Daily Journal – Day 73

| Date: |
| Weight: |
| Strengths: |
| |
| |
| |
| Weaknesses: |
| |
| |
| |
| Notes (how you felt, what influenced food choices, exercise/weights time, etc.): |

Today you can see where the changes you need to make to keep control of the Yeast Beast are simple: control the Yeast foods and move more. Consider your exercise program work out a routine that you can live with and possibly enjoy.

Daily Journal – Day 74

Date:
Weight:
Strengths:
Weaknesses:
Notes (how you felt, what influenced food choices, exercise/weights time, etc.):

You're still in the danger zone; this is where the yo-yo starts. Fight the Yeast Beast! No Yeast foods today; try to eat lightly today or get an extra few minutes of exercise.

Daily Journal – Day 75

Date:
Weight:
Strengths:
Weaknesses:
Notes (how you felt, what influenced food choices, exercise/weights time, etc.):

Controlling the Yeast Beast is a big step in reclaiming your life; you do not need to be overweight or obese; get control today for every day. *Mirror, Mirror on the wall…* spend some extra time with the mirror.

Daily Journal – Day 76

Date:
Weight:
Strengths:
Weaknesses:
Notes (how you felt, what influenced food choices, exercise/weights time, etc.):

Are you getting frustrated or feel that things are going too slowly? The Yeast Beast makes chemicals which are toxic to you. The Yeast Beast has been in control for a long time and will not give up easily. *Every day is a battle in the war with the Beast. Today I will win today's battle.*

Daily Journal – Day 77

Date:	
Weight:	
Strengths:	

Weaknesses:

Notes (how you felt, what influenced food choices, exercise/weights time, etc.):

You are fighting a lonely battle with the Beast and many people cannot understand. Be patient with those around you; most of all be patient with yourself.

Daily Journal – Day 78

Date:
Weight:
Strengths:
Weaknesses:
Notes (how you felt, what influenced food choices, exercise/weights time, etc.):

The Yeast Beast is the cause of obesity. Fight the Beast and avoid a lot of health problems. *I want to age in a healthy manner. I will do today what will make ma healthy for my tomorrows.*

Daily Journal – Day 79

Date:
Weight:
Strengths:
Weaknesses:
Notes (how you felt, what influenced food choices, exercise/weights time, etc.):

I really lost 180 pounds without surgery or liposuction; so can you. Fight the Yeast Beast as if your life depended on it. It does.

Daily Journal – Day 80

Date:	
Weight:	
Strengths:	

Weaknesses:

Notes (how you felt, what influenced food choices, exercise/weights time, etc.):

Without a Gastrointestinal bypass or Liposuction you will have a better old age. Save your money: get fit.

Daily Journal – Day 81

Date:	
Weight:	
Strengths:	
Weaknesses:	

Notes (how you felt, what influenced food choices, exercise/weights time, etc.):

The Yeast Beast makes your weight go back up; you *MUST* control the Yeast Beast for any diet to be ultimately successful, with longevity.

Daily Journal – Day 82

Date:	
Weight:	
Strengths:	

Weaknesses:

Notes (how you felt, what influenced food choices, exercise/weights time, etc.):

Obesity Recovery = Controlling the Yeast Beast & Losing The Weight

Daily Journal – Day 83

Date:	
Weight:	
Strengths:	
Weaknesses:	

Notes (how you felt, what influenced food choices, exercise/weights time, etc.):

Obesity Rehabilitation is the physical restoration to good condition, operation, or capacity of a sick or disabled person by therapeutic measures and reeducation to full participation in the activities of a normal life. *Obesity is a disease, caused by the yeast Beast. I am getting well.*

Daily Journal – Day 84

Date:
Weight:
Strengths:
Weaknesses:
Notes (how you felt, what influenced food choices, exercise/weights time, etc.):

Motion of any type: walking with weights, dancing or a work out machine. Get moving; it is your life. Being overweight takes a heavy (no pun intended) toll on you. Get your health back today; keep fighting the Yeast Beast today. *Every battle day with the Beast I win is a day closer to winning the war.*

Daily Journal – Day 85

Date:	
Weight:	
Strengths:	
Weaknesses:	

Notes (how you felt, what influenced food choices, exercise/weights time, etc.):

Yeast in a healthy body is usually commensal. If you are healthy, the right size and weight, the correct BMI, can perform a sustained (20-30 minute) high-performance workout, and have never taken broad-spectrum antibiotic treatment, the micro flora in your body is probably balanced. This is not you; do not miss a day of your anti-fungals.

Daily Journal – Day 86

Date:	
Weight:	
Strengths:	
Weaknesses:	

Notes (how you felt, what influenced food choices, exercise/weights time, etc.):

Still in the danger zone; the last time you got this far or close you fed the Beast and blew up again. Don't let it happen again; this time, fight the Beast.

Daily Journal – Day 87

Date:	
Weight:	
Strengths:	
Weaknesses:	

Notes (how you felt, what influenced food choices, exercise/weights time, etc.):

Love exercise just a little more than you love to eat and you will control the Yeast Beast. OK, maybe you will never love exercise, but you can love how it helps you keep the Beast and the fat away. *Movement keeps my body limber and my metabolism higher. The harder I move, the longer I move, the healthier I will be.*

Daily Journal – Day 88

Date:	
Weight:	
Strengths:	
Weaknesses:	

Notes (how you felt, what influenced food choices, exercise/weights time, etc.):

You brush your teeth every day; take your anti-fungals every morning and fighting the Yeast Beast will be on automatic.

Daily Journal – Day 89

Date:
Weight:
Strengths:
Weaknesses:
Notes (how you felt, what influenced food choices, exercise/weights time, etc.):

As the weight comes off, strengthen your commitment to motion. Whatever your program is, keep moving get limber and you will have a better old age.

Daily Journal – Day 90

Date:
Weight:
Strengths:
Weaknesses:
Notes (how you felt, what influenced food choices, exercise/weights time, etc.):

Today is the ¾ mark in this battle with the Yeast Beast. Renew your commitment; do something extra to beat the Beast today. How are you doing on your chosen diet? Remember you can change diets, but not more often than once a month. Work to find what diet suits your body and personality.

Daily Journal – Day 91

Date:
Weight:
Strengths:
Weaknesses:
Notes (how you felt, what influenced food choices, exercise/weights time, etc.):

The last 30 days and you will beat the Yeast Beast. It is your life; do not give up.

Daily Journal – Day 92

Date:	
Weight:	
Strengths:	
Weaknesses:	

Notes (how you felt, what influenced food choices, exercise/weights time, etc.):

The Yeast Beast has given you unwanted weight in the past; as you drop the weight laugh at the Yeast Beast. In fact, laugh out loud and hard; the shaking of your innards is beneficial to your heart and digestion.

Daily Journal – Day 93

Date:
Weight:
Strengths:
Weaknesses:
Notes (how you felt, what influenced food choices, exercise/weights time, etc.):

You are still fighting the Yeast Beast and you are winning; take your anti-fungals and keep winning. It's your life. Spend some extra time in the mirror today.

Daily Journal – Day 94

Date:	
Weight:	
Strengths:	

Weaknesses:

Notes (how you felt, what influenced food choices, exercise/weights time, etc.):

Look to yourself for the reinforcement you need; find strength inside if you to beat the Beast. *I am in control of my body. The Beast will not drag me back down.*

Daily Journal – Day 95

Date:
Weight:
Strengths:
Weaknesses:
Notes (how you felt, what influenced food choices, exercise/weights time, etc.):

The Yeast Beast is a bully and very sneaky; fight the Yeast Beast with every bite you take.

Daily Journal – Day 96

Date:	
Weight:	
Strengths:	

Weaknesses:

Notes (how you felt, what influenced food choices, exercise/weights time, etc.):

The Yeast Beast knows you are serious now and it will get ugly; when that late night craving or mood swing hits, take a deep breath (in fact take several) and laugh at the Yeast Beast and the craving will go away.

Daily Journal – Day 97

Date:	
Weight:	
Strengths:	

Weaknesses:

Notes (how you felt, what influenced food choices, exercise/weights time, etc.):

As you experiment with different foods, notice how your body reacts. Introduce new foods slowly and individually. Identify your most favorite, and most likely 'illegal', foods; save these for well deserved splurges, and keep your splurges far apart and in small quantity. *I eat to live; I don't live to eat.*

Daily Journal – Day 98

Date:	
Weight:	
Strengths:	
Weaknesses:	

Notes (how you felt, what influenced food choices, exercise/weights time, etc.):

Do something really nice for someone who has been supportive to you. Thank them for helping you win this war; seriously: let them know it is a war.

Daily Journal – Day 99

Date:	
Weight:	
Strengths:	
Weaknesses:	

Notes (how you felt, what influenced food choices, exercise/weights time, etc.):

When was the last time you stepped up your exercise? Getting that blood circulating and moving those muscles raises your metabolism, which helps you lose weight faster, even when sleeping! Step up your exercise every time you start getting comfortable.

Daily Journal – Day 100

Date:
Weight:
Strengths:
Weaknesses:
Notes (how you felt, what influenced food choices, exercise/weights time, etc.):

100 days and you are beating the Yeast Beast and on your way to a better life; keep beating on the Yeast Beast. Have you taken photos lately?

Daily Journal – Day 101

Date:
Weight:
Strengths:
Weaknesses:
Notes (how you felt, what influenced food choices, exercise/weights time, etc.):

Time to review your journal and photos again. Where are you now from where you started? How much weight have you lost, and how much do you want to lose? If you have been serious about this program, you have the Beast under control now.

Daily Journal – Day 102

Date:
Weight:
Strengths:
Weaknesses:
Notes (how you felt, what influenced food choices, exercise/weights time, etc.):

We create much of our own experience, both by desire and design. Our 'filters', the way we choose to see things, play an important part in this. Look at your filters; are they positive? Are they self supporting? *Happy is as happy <u>says</u> it is.*

Daily Journal – Day 103

Date:
Weight:
Strengths:
Weaknesses:
Notes (how you felt, what influenced food choices, exercise/weights time, etc.):

Have you had a play day in your closet yet? Get *RID* of all the clothes that are at least a full size too big. You are never going back there!

Daily Journal – Day 104

Date:	
Weight:	
Strengths:	

Weaknesses:

Notes (how you felt, what influenced food choices, exercise/weights time, etc.):

Fat comes on in layers around the body, and comes off in reverse order. The fat that came on first will be the last to go.

Daily Journal – Day 105

Date:	
Weight:	
Strengths:	

Weaknesses:

Notes (how you felt, what influenced food choices, exercise/weights time, etc.):

You are in the final stretch of the Yeast war; in fact, if you have been faithful to the program, at this point you're micro flora is probably balanced by now. If you have no urges, you can start weaning yourself from the anti-fungals. Keep taking the probiotics!

Daily Journal – Day 106

Date:
Weight:
Strengths:
Weaknesses:
Notes (how you felt, what influenced food choices, exercise/weights time, etc.):

In these last two weeks, it's time to gather all your data, analyze what works best for you, and start creating your own program to continue the weight loss. Start looking at how you'd like your program to lay out: realistically, how much weight do you have to lose and how long do you think you should take to lose it?

Daily Journal – Day 107

Date:
Weight:
Strengths:
Weaknesses:
Notes (how you felt, what influenced food choices, exercise/weights time, etc.):

The important thing to remember is that the Yeast Beast is a resident of your body. In control, it's not a bad thing. But when the resident starts spreading out on all the property you own, it's dangerous to you.

Daily Journal – Day 108

Date:
Weight:
Strengths:
Weaknesses:
Notes (how you felt, what influenced food choices, exercise/weights time, etc.):

Today put on 1- something new, 2- something you haven't worn in years, and 3- something you wore three months ago. Do it all in the mirror.

Daily Journal – Day 109

Date:
Weight:
Strengths:
Weaknesses:
Notes (how you felt, what influenced food choices, exercise/weights time, etc.):

How much weight did you need to lose when you started? Whether 50 or 250 pounds, you should have a great idea now of how much food control and how much movement control you need to keep the pounds coming off.

Daily Journal – Day 110

Date:
Weight:
Strengths:
Weaknesses:
Notes (how you felt, what influenced food choices, exercise/weights time, etc.):

Exercise legalizes cheating. If you are going to cheat, work out extra in relation to how big a cheat it is. The key to successful cheating is to move more and to cheat infrequently and in small amounts. I try to do the extra exercise *first* so it doesn't become a broken promise; the cheat is more enjoyable if you don't owe on it later.

Daily Journal – Day 111

Date:
Weight:
Strengths:
Weaknesses:
Notes (how you felt, what influenced food choices, exercise/weights time, etc.):

Are you saying affirmations? Use the ones in the journal or make up your own, but do try to say something positive and reinforcing to yourself in the mirror each day.

Daily Journal – Day 112

Date:
Weight:
Strengths:
Weaknesses:
Notes (how you felt, what influenced food choices, exercise/weights time, etc.):

Review your journal today looking specifically at one item; tomorrow and the next day do the same, using a different focus. *I realize I used to always _____ but now I _____.*

Daily Journal – Day 113

Date:
Weight:
Strengths:
Weaknesses:
Notes (how you felt, what influenced food choices, exercise/weights time, etc.):

If you haven't done so in the last few weeks, go get a haircut. Get brave and let your stylist do something different, or get *really* brave and go to someone who never knew you heavier and has no preconceived concept of how your hair should look.

Daily Journal – Day 114

Date:	
Weight:	
Strengths:	

Weaknesses:

Notes (how you felt, what influenced food choices, exercise/weights time, etc.):

This is the last week of this journal. I hope you are still writing. Take some time to write down the insights you have gotten from your journal.

Daily Journal – Day 115

Date:	
Weight:	
Strengths:	
Weaknesses:	
Notes (how you felt, what influenced food choices, exercise/weights time, etc.):	

Don't ever forget the Beast is merely at bay. Like the little beasts in *Gremlins*, it can raise its ugly head any time you feed it wrong. Stick to your diet and your exercise program to lose weight, and keep taking your probiotics. Do anti-fungals for 30 days every three months. Never let the Beast control you again!

Daily Journal – Day 116

Date:	
Weight:	
Strengths:	
Weaknesses:	

Notes (how you felt, what influenced food choices, exercise/weights time, etc.):

If you've found the journal helpful, consider going to a stationary or book store for a bound journal; they have them from cheap to outrageously expensive. Treat yourself to one that pleases you. Make it your journal for the next few months.

Daily Journal – Day 117

Date:
Weight:
Strengths:
Weaknesses:
Notes (how you felt, what influenced food choices, exercise/weights time, etc.):

What did the scale say this morning? Most importantly, what did *how you felt* when you got up this morning tell you? What does the mirror tell you? Take stock of the ways your progress to date has affected your life in the last 100+ days.

Daily Journal – Day 119

Date:	
Weight:	
Strengths:	

Weaknesses:

Notes (how you felt, what influenced food choices, exercise/weights time, etc.):

You can stop taking the anti-fungals now; mark your calendar to begin taking them again in 90 days. Take one kind for thirty days; next time you detox, use a different anti-fungal. You can alternate or rotate them.

Daily Journal – Day 120

Date:
Weight:
Strengths:
Weaknesses:
Notes (how you felt, what influenced food choices, exercise/weights time, etc.):

You made it!! 120 days and you should be Yeast Beast infestation free, and considerably thinner. Please take time to drop me a line and share your progress. I hope you stay with it until you reach *Fairy Tale* status. Good luck!
beauty@beautyandtheyeastbeast.com